Statistical Problems in Genetics and Molecular Biology

Statistical Problems in Genetics and Molecular Biology

Norman Drinkwater and Carter Denniston

An enlightened one
Perceives without reflection
Ponders without words.

Carter Denniston
English Haiku and Other Poems (2005)

TABLE OF CONTENTS

FOREWORD

Carter Denniston, a Tribute

The original intent for this book was that Norman Drinkwater and Carter Denniston be co-authors. Unfortunately, this was prevented by Denniston's premature death. Carter was greatly influential in the development of the book and it is appropriate that his contribution be appreciated and that he be remembered.

Carter Denniston was born in Milwaukee in 1938. I first met him when he was principal violist in the Wisconsin University orchestra. Yes, he was a gifted musician and went through the University on a music scholarship. He majored in anthropology where his teaching skills, evident throughout his academic life, were first appreciated. He won his first teaching award as a graduate assistant in anthropology. Later he changed his major to genetics, became my student, and received his Ph.D. in 1968. Two years later he joined the Genetics faculty where he spent the rest of his life.

It was as a graduate student that Carter's ability in logical analysis became apparent. He came under the influence of Charles Cotterman, from whom he acquired his taste for finite mathematics and combinatorics. His work was complex and difficult. He extended Cotterman's K coefficients to multiple alleles and multiple loci with linkage, a major feat. Although he was formally my student his major influence was Cotterman and he retained his interests in this area for the rest of his life.

Carter liked to teach, did it well, and did far more than his share. He also was active in committee work, both in the University and nationally. He collaborated in research projects, often as a statistical consultant, with researchers who appreciated his thoroughness, his logical rigor, and his depth of scholarship.

Carter and his wife, Glenda, enjoyed outdoor wilderness-type activities. As graduate students they jointly studied the Alaskan Inuits. For several years they volunteered to participate in an ophthalmological team in the Philippines. It is evident that Carter's interests and activities were broad and varied and that he had a social conscience.

He loved number theory and had looked forward to retirement as an opportunity to engage in this on a full-time basis. Alas it was not to be.

Shortly after retiring, he was struck down by cancer and died on September 27, 2005. He never had a chance to pursue his favorite subject.

James F. Crow
November, 2011

PREFACE

This book evolved from the notes for a course of the same title that we've taught for the last eighteen years at the University of Wisconsin to graduate students in cancer biology, genetics, molecular biology, and other biomedical programs. We began teaching that course to counter the notion held by (some) molecular biologists that, "if you need statistics to analyze your data, you should have done a better experiment." We hope to convince you that by considering the statistical issues inherent in your research, you will be able to design better experiments and develop a sense of the degree of confidence you can place in the conclusions you draw from your studies.

Part of the antipathy biologists have for statistics arises from the way statistical analysis is taught in many introductory courses. Generally, the focus of these courses is on statistical methods for analysis of continuous random variables that follow explicit, well-defined models. In contrast, the nature of the variation that underlies most of the experiments we do as biologists is difficult to specify in detail. We will concentrate on a class of statistical methods, so-called nonparametric statistics, which requires us to make very few assumptions regarding the model that gives rise to the data. These methods are also attractive because they are usually simple to apply and have considerable intuitive appeal.

The first section of the book will review basic probability theory and general considerations for hypothesis testing. Both of these topics are covered in detail in most introductory statistics books. An excellent recent statistics text with a biological focus is "Biometry," by Robert A. Sokal and F. James Rohlf (Freeman, 1995).

For the material on nonparametric statistics, we recommend the following texts or monographs:

"Practical Nonparametric Statistics," by W. J. Conover (Wiley, third ed., 1999), provides an accessible and reasonably comprehensive text for this subject.

"Nonparametric Statistical Methods," by Myles Hollander and Douglas A. Wolfe (Wiley, second ed., 1999) is more methodologically oriented, with explicit instructions on performing a variety of statistical tests and many examples, but is harder to follow on the theory of the tests. This book also has extensive tables for the statistics described in this course.

"Nonparametrics: Statistical Methods based on Ranks," by E. L. Lehman (Prentice Hall, 1998), is a more advanced and theoretically oriented monograph. Much of the material presented below on extension of the methods to the complications of multiple comparisons, multiple experiments and confounding variables is developed from Lehman's treatment of these subjects.

"Categorical Data Analysis," by Alan Agresti (Wiley, 2002), provides a comprehensive treatment of its subject. The same author has also published "An Introduction to Categorical Data Analysis," (Wiley, 2007), which is a more accessible introduction to the field.

More detailed discussions and the original references for the statistical tests described in Chapters 5 through 8 can be found in either the Conover, Hollander and Wolfe, or Agresti texts. Nearly all of the methods described in this book can be performed using the *Mstat* program developed by one of us (ND). A copy of the User Manual for the most recent version (5.5) of the software is included as Appendix 7.

As noted above, much of the material in this book grew out of a course that I taught with Carter Denniston from 1994 to 2004. I enjoyed that decade of teaching with Carter enormously and learned a great deal from him about teaching well. I particularly miss both his dry sense of humor and knack for analogies that stick in students' minds. We lost Carter too soon when he died at the age of 67 in 2005. His friend and colleague, James F. Crow, provides a tribute to Carter in the foreword to this book.

I want to express my gratitude to many colleagues who provided critical advice, encouragement, and sample data over the years. In particular, to Bill Engels, who developed a predecessor to this course with me from 1986-1992, and to James F. Crow, Andrea Bilger, and Bill Sugden. Thanks are also due to the generations of students who made it very clear when I was, or wasn't, getting the point across.

Norman Drinkwater

1. SETS, COMBINATORICS & PROBABILITY

The following constitutes a basic introduction to sets, combinatorics, and probability necessary for competent statistical analysis. The examples we use will be heavy on genetics because of our own research interests. Read this chapter carefully and try the problems; then use it as a reference for the rest of the course.

1.1. Sets

We introduce the idea of a set here only because it is often helpful to think of **events** as sets, and it is of events that we calculate probabilities. For example, from a mating of type *Aa* × *Aa* there are three possible offspring: *AA*, *Aa* and *aa*–a set, or sample space, of three elements. Any event concerning this one mating can be expressed as a subset of this set of three primitive events, *e.g.*, the event "*A_*" is represented by the set (*AA*, *Aa*), the event "homozygote" is represented by (*AA*, *aa*). In practically all of the problems we encounter, the sample space will consist of a finite number of primitive events, and any event we can imagine will correspond to a subset of that sample space.

Examples 1.1

A. Suppose the mating *Aa* x *Aa* produces three children. Then the sample space consists of 27 events. Note, here, the primitive events are themselves sets.

AA,AA,AA	AA,Aa,AA	AA,aa,AA	Aa,AA,AA
Aa,Aa,AA	Aa,aa,AA	aa,AA,AA	aa,Aa,AA
aa,aa,AA	AA,AA,Aa	AA,Aa,Aa	AA,aa,Aa
Aa,AA,Aa	Aa,Aa,Aa	Aa,aa,Aa	aa,AA,Aa
aa,Aa,Aa	aa,aa,Aa	AA,AA,aa	AA,Aa,aa
AA,aa,aa	Aa,AA,aa	Aa,Aa,aa	Aa,aa,aa
aa,AA,aa	aa,Aa,aa	aa,aa,aa	

The event "at least two recessive children" is the set {*aa,aa,AA*; *aa,AA,aa*; *AA,aa,aa*; *aa,aa,Aa*; *aa,Aa,aa*; *Aa,aa,aa*; *aa,aa,aa*}. The event "the first child is *AA*" comprises nine of the primitive events, and the event "the second child is a homozygote" comprises 18 of the primitive events. Any event imaginable may be represented by some subset of these 27 primitive events. How many are there? Answer: $2^{27}-1=134,217,727$.

B. Consider a sequence of six bases (nucleotides). There are $4^6 = 4096$ such sequences (we won't display them!). The event "AANNTT", where N denotes any base, represents a set comprising 16 of these sequences.

1.1.1. Set.

A set is simply a collection of objects. No order is implied. An object included in a set is said to belong to that set and to be an element of the set. The elements of a set can be anything, even other sets.

Example 1.2

Let the set A = {Mike, the moon, a particular loaf of bread, the set of integers greater than -1}. This set contains four elements, one of which is, itself, a set containing a countable infinity of elements.

There are two ways of defining a particular set. The first is simply to enumerate its elements as we did for set A, above. The second is to characterize the elements in some way, for example, let B = {$x|x$ is a female}. This statement is read: "B consists of all organisms, x, such that x is a female." That is, B is the set of all females.

1.1.2. Union.

The union of two sets, A and B, written $A \cup B$, is the set of all elements belonging either to A or to B or to both.

Examples 1.3

A. The union of the set {a,b,c} and the set {b,c,d,e} is {a,b,c,d,e}.

B. Consider the mating *Aa* x *aa*. The set of all possible families of size three is X ={(*Aa,Aa,Aa*), (*Aa,Aa,aa*), (*Aa,aa,Aa*), (*aa,Aa,Aa*), (*Aa,aa,aa*), (*aa,Aa,aa*), (*aa,aa,Aa*), (*aa,aa,aa*)}. The set of all such families in which the first child is *aa* is Y = {(*aa,Aa,Aa*), (*aa,Aa,aa*), (*aa,aa,Aa*), (*aa,aa,aa*)} and the set of all such families in which the first two children are *aa* is Z={(*aa,aa,Aa*), (*aa,aa,aa*)}. In this case, the union of Y and Z is just Y.

C. Considering our six-base sequences, again—the set "AACNTT" = (AACCTT, AACGTT, AACATT, AACTTT) and the set "AANCTT" = (AACCTT, AAGCTT, AAACTT, AATCTT). The union "AACNTT" ∪ "AANCTT" = (AACCTT, AACGTT, AACATT, AACTTT, AAGCTT, AAACTT, AATCTT).

Note that union corresponds to the English word "or" in the inclusive sense. Throughout this book, we will usually write "A or B" rather than "A ∪ B" when A and B refer to events.

1.1.3. Complement.

The complement of a set, A, written A^c, is the set of all elements not belonging to A. Our use of complement arises from the helpful fact that it is sometimes the case that to find the probability of an event, A, it is easier to calculate [1 - (the probability of the complement of A)] than the probability of A, itself.

Examples 1.4

A. The P{of at least one girl in a family of five children} = 1 - P{of no girls in a family of five children}.

B. In families of size six from the mating *Aa* x *aa*, the event "at least two *aa* children" (the union of four events) is the complement of the event "less than two *aa* children" (the union of two events).

C. For our six-base sequences, the complement of the set "ANNNNN" is the set (CNNNNN, GNNNNN, TNNNNN).

1.1.4. Intersection.

The intersection of two sets, A and B, written $A \cap B$, is the set of all elements belonging to both A and B.

Examples 1.5

A. The intersection of the sets N={b,c,d,e,g} and P={a,c,e,g,h} is the set N∩P={c,e,g}.

B. The intersection of the sets Y and Z, in Example 1.3.B, is Z.

C. The intersection of the sets M={x|x is a male} and F={x|x is a female} is empty.

D. The set "AACNTT" ∩ "AANCTT" = the set (AACCTT).

Note that intersection corresponds to the English word "and". We will often write "A and B" or just "AB" to denote intersection.

1.1.5. Subset.

A set, A, is said to be a subset of the set, B, written $A \subseteq B$, if every element of A is also an element of B. Z was a subset of Y, in the Example 1.3.B.

1.1.6. Some properties of union and intersection.

For any three sets, A, B and C:

$$AB = BA \qquad\qquad A(BC) = (AB)C$$
$$A \cup B = B \cup A \qquad\qquad A \cup (B \cup C) = (A \cup B) \cup C$$
$$A \cap (B \cup C) = AB \cup AC \qquad\qquad (A \cup B) \cap (A \cup C) = A \cup BC$$

DeMorgan's Rules:
$$(A \cup B)^c = (A^c)(B^c) \qquad\qquad (AB)^c = (A^c) \cup (B^c)$$

The operations of union and intersection have some of the properties of addition and multiplication. Note certain peculiarities, however. For example, $A \cap (A \cup B) = A \cup AB = A$. You can convince yourself of the truth of these various equalities by studying the Venn diagram, below.

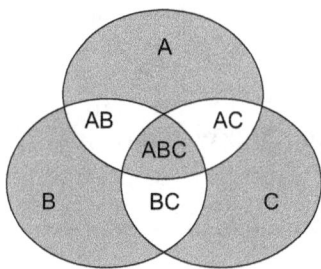

The rules also apply to the truth value of statements. For example, if you let A="physicians are wise" and B="professors are stupid", and so forth, all the rules apply.

1.2. Combinatorics

To calculate probabilities we will often be required to determine all possible results of a particular experiment. The following "rules of counting" will be helpful.

1.2.1. Rule of sum.

If event X can happen in x different ways and a distinct event Y can happen in y different ways, then the event "X or Y" can happen in $(x + y)$ ways.

Examples 1.6

A. For an X-linked locus with two alleles, a woman can be any of three genotypes, a man any of two. A random individual (sex unspecified) can be any of five genotypes.

B. The event "AANTTT" or "AAANTT" can happen in 7 ways. Why doesn't the rule work here?

C. A menu lists six entrees, five desserts, and three salads. How many ways can I order an entree or a salad? Answer: 6+3.

1.2.2. Rule of product.

If event X can happen in x ways and a distinct event Y can happen in y ways, then the event "X and Y" can happen in xy ways.

Example 1.7

For an X-linked locus with two alleles, a woman can be any of three genotypes, a man any of two. A couple can then be any of six pairs of genotypes. This is the "menu" rule: *e.g.*, if there are 6 entrees and 5 desserts, there are 30 possible meals. Notice that this extends to more than two selections. If there are, in addition, 7 appetizers to choose from, the total number of different meals is 210.

1.2.3. Power set.

Any set of n elements has 2^n subsets. The set of all subsets of a set is called its power set. A power set thus has 2^n elements.

Example 1.8

If A = {a,b,c}, the power set of A is the set {∅, a, b, c, ab, ac, bc, abc}. "∅", here, denotes the empty set. It is a convention that the power set includes as one of its elements the empty set, the set containing no element. An example: How many sounds can you make on a piano with 88 keys? Answer: $2^{88} - 1$. We don't count the empty set here because it represents no sound!

1.2.4. Permutations.

A permutation is an ordered arrangement. The number of permutations of n distinct objects is

$$n! = n(n-1)(n-2)(n-3)...(2)(1).$$

Examples 1.9

A. The number of permutations of the three letters, a, b and c, is six: abc, acb, bac, bca, cab, cba.

B. Consider a chromosome containing five loci, *A, B, C, D,* and *E*, on its long arm. There are 5! = 120 possible maps (orders) for these loci.

1.2.5. Ordered selections.

The number of ordered selections of r things out of n distinct objects is

$$(n)_r = n(n-1)(n-2)...(n-r+1) = \frac{n!}{(n-r)!}$$

Examples 1.10

A. The number of ordered pairs that can be gotten from the set {a, b, c} is six: ab, ba, ac, ca, bc, cb.

B. Eight students wish to see you next Thursday, but you have only five times free. The number of different appointment schedules possible for that day, assuming you use all your time slots, is 8×7×6×5×4 = 6720.

1.2.6. Unordered selections (binomial coefficients).

The number of ways r things can be chosen out of n distinct objects (regardless of order) is

$$\binom{n}{r} = \frac{(n)_r}{r!} = \frac{n!}{r!(n-r)!}$$

These are sometimes called "combination numbers" because they give the number of combinations (unordered selections) of size r that can be made from a set of size n.

Examples 1.11

A. If there are n alleles at a locus, the number of heterozygotes possible is $\binom{n}{2} = n(n-1)/2$.

The number of homozygotes is n, so the total number of genotypes is $n(n-1)/2 + n = n(n+1)/2$.

B. With respect to the scheduling problem in Example 1.10, you can pick five of the eight students to see on Thursday in $\binom{8}{5} = 56$ ways and given the chosen five, there are $5! = 120$ ways to schedule them. The product is $56 \times 120 = 6720$, as before.

C. In how many ways can an RNA molecule of 10 bases be constructed with 3 U, 3 G, 3 A, and 1 C?

Answer: $\binom{10}{3}\binom{7}{3}\binom{4}{3}\binom{1}{1} = \dfrac{10!}{3!3!3!1!}$

Note that $\binom{n}{r} = \binom{n-1}{r} + \binom{n-1}{r-1}$, $\binom{1}{0} = 1$, and $\binom{1}{1} = 1$, which lead to the familiar Pascal's triangle

```
                              1
                    1                   1
              1           2           1
         1          3           3          1
     1         4           6          4          1
  1         5         10          10          5          1
                              ...
```

1.2.7. Multinomial coefficients.

The number of ways that a set of n objects can be divided into k distinguishable parts of which the first contains r_1 objects, the second r_2 objects, and so on ($r_1+r_2+...+r_k = n$) is

$$\binom{n}{r_1 r_2 ... r_k} = \frac{n!}{r_1! r_2! ... r_k!}$$

Example 1.12

From a mating of type *Aa* x *Aa*, four children are produced: 2 *AA*, 1 *Aa* and 1 *aa*. How many different birth orders are possible? The answer is 4!/2!1!1! = 12. Let 1=*AA*, 2=*Aa* and 3=*aa*. The 12 orders are: 1123, 1132, 1213, 1312, 1231, 1321, 2113, 3112, 2131, 3121, 2311, 3211.

1.3. Probability

One can often think of probabilities as proportions. For example, to ask "what is the probability that a randomly selected person is a heterozygote?" is simply to ask "what proportion of all persons are heterozygotes?" Often a probability is thought of as the proportion of times an event will occur *in the long run*, in a series of repeated "experiments". For example, consider the simple pedigree below.

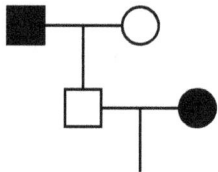

A normal man whose father is an albino marries an albino woman. What is the risk of albinism to their child? The prospective father is definitely a heterozygote. The risk to the child is therefore one-half. By this we mean that in a large series of families just like this one, each producing a child, in the long run about half of the children will be albino and half will be normal. We are forced to think of this particular family as a member of a larger group of families in which the proportion of affected children is expected to be one-half. The larger group may not even exist except in our imagination. If it did exist, and we told each of the families that their child will be albino, we would be correct half the time and incorrect the other half *in the long run*.

The above view of probability is not without its problems. The concept of *in the long run* is not easy to define in a precise manner. One version of this approach is to say that the probability of an event, E, is said to be p, if as the sample size, n, gets larger the observed proportion of cases of E, p_E, approaches p in the sense that

$$\Pr(\,|p_E - p| > e) \to 0 \text{ for any } e \text{ as } n \to \infty.$$

This is, of course, hopelessly circular, because we are assuming the concept of probability to define it.

The interpretation of probability described above is usually called *objective* probability or *frequentist* probability. An alternative interpretation is that probability is simply a measure of belief; this is known as *subjective* or *personal* probability. For example, suppose I claim that the probability that Hillary Clinton will run for President in 2016 is 0.6. That is an expression of my conviction that she will run. It is difficult—perhaps impossible—to think of Clinton embedded in a series of possible election campaigns among which she runs 60% of times and demurs 40%.

1.3.1. Probabilities are normed.

For any event, E, $0 \le P(E) \le 1$.

Example 1.13

An event with Pr = 1 must happen. An event with Pr = 0 cannot happen.

1.3.2. The Pr of the union of two events.

For any two events, E_1 and E_2, the probability of their union is

$$P(E_1 \text{ or } E_2) = P(E_1) + P(E_2) - P(E_1 E_2).$$

Example 1.14

Consider a mating of type $Aa \times aa$. Let E_1 be the event that the first child is aa and let E_2 be the event that the second child is aa. What is the probability of the event "E_1 or E_2", that either child is aa? It is

$$P(E_1) + P(E_2) - P(E_1 E_2) = 1/2 + 1/2 - 1/4 = 3/4.$$

Note that this is 1 - P(neither is aa) = 1-P(both are Aa)
$$= P(\text{at least one is } aa).$$

There are often multiple ways of expressing the same event.

If two events, E_1 and E_2, are mutually exclusive, that is, their intersection is empty ($E_1 E_2 = \varnothing$) and therefore the Pr of their intersection is zero ($P[E_1 E_2] = 0$), then we have

$$P(E_1 \text{ or } E_2) = P(E_1) + P(E_2), \text{ as a special case.}$$

Example 1.15

The probability that a child from the mating $Aa \times Aa$ is either AA or Aa is, from our general rule: P(AA or Aa)= P(AA) + P(Aa) - P(AA and Aa); but the last term is clearly zero because the two events AA and Aa are mutually exclusive (also called 'disjoint'). A child cannot be both. So P(*AA* or *Aa*) = 1/4 + 1/2 = 3/4.

1.3.3. The Pr of the union of more than two events.

Let Σ denote summation. The union of n events is

$$P(E_1 \text{ or } E_2 \text{ or ... or } E_n) = \Sigma P(E_i) - \Sigma P(E_i E_j) + \Sigma P(E_i E_j E_k) -$$

$$... -(-1)^n P(E_1 E_2 ... E_n).$$

For three events we have

$$P(A \text{ or } B \text{ or } C) = P(A)+P(B)+P(C)-P(AB)-P(AC)-P(BC)+P(ABC)$$

This formula can easily be understood by reference to the Venn diagram in section 1.1.6.

Example 1.16

Consider, again, the *Aa* x *aa* mating. What is the probability that either the first child or the second child or the third child is *aa*? Let A= first child is *aa*, B=second child is *aa*, and C=third child is *aa*. Then P(A or B or C) = 1/2 + 1/2 + 1/2 - 1/4 - 1/4 - 1/4 + 1/8 = 7/8. This is, of course, 1 - P(all are *Aa*).

1.3.4. Conditional probability.

The conditional probability of E_1 given E_2 is defined as

$$P(E_1|E_2) = \frac{P(E_1 E_2)}{P(E_2)}$$

In words, we are asking: In those cases in which E_2 has occurred, in what proportion has E_1 also occurred?

Examples 1.17

A. From the mating $Aa \times Aa$ a child is born with the dominant phenotype. What is the Pr the child is Aa?

$$P(Aa|A\_) = P(Aa \text{ and } A\_)/P(A\_)$$
$$= P(Aa)/P(A\_) = (1/2)/(3/4) = 2/3.$$

B. If the population is in Hardy-Weinberg equilibrium (*i.e.*, randomly mating), what proportion of $A\_$ individuals are heterozygotes?

Answer: $\dfrac{2q}{1+q}$ where q is the frequency of the a allele.

C. What is the Pr that a random oligo containing five bases has 2 U's given that it has at least one?

Answer: $\dfrac{\binom{5}{2}(1/4)^2(3/4)^3}{1-(3/4)^5} = \dfrac{\binom{5}{2}3^3}{4^5-3^5}$

1.3.5. Writing an intersection in terms of conditionals.

This rule is sometimes very helpful in calculating probabilities. The following is true for any set of events $E_1, E_2, \ldots, E_n$.

$$P(E_1E_2\ldots E_n) = P(E_1)P(E_2|E_1)P(E_3|E_1E_2) \ldots P(E_n|E_1E_2\ldots E_{n-1}).$$

Here, the numbering of the events is arbitrary; any permutation of the subscripts $(1,2,\ldots,n)$ will work as well.

Examples 1.18

A. Suppose A = male, B = unfaithful, C = married. We can write

$$P(ABC) = P(A)P(B|A)P(C|AB) = P(A)P(C|A)P(B|AC)$$

$$= P(B)P(A|B)P(C|AB) = P(B)P(C|B)P(A|BC)$$

$$= P(C)P(A|C)P(B|AC) = P(C)P(B|C)P(A|BC).$$

Think about the meaning of each expression in words.

B. Another example more germane to human genetics: Suppose you want to know the P(parents are both *Aa* | child is *aa*). From the definition of conditional probability we may write this as P(parents are both *Aa* and the child is *aa*)/P(child is *aa*). The numerator can then be written as P(parents are both *Aa*)P(child is *aa* | parents are both *Aa*), by our rule, which is easier to calculate because it involves a simple Mendelian segregation frequency (1/4). Thus , if the frequency of the *A* gene is p =1-q and we assume Hardy-Weinberg equilibrium we get
P(parents both *Aa* | child is *aa*) =

$$\frac{P(\text{parents both } Aa)P(\text{Child is } aa \,|\, \text{parents both } Aa)}{P(\text{child is } aa)}$$

$$= \frac{4p^2q^2 \times (1/4)}{q^2} = p^2$$

1.3.6. Independence.

Two events E_1 and E_2 are said to be independent if $P(E_1E_2)=P(E_1)P(E_2)$ or what amounts to the same thing, if $P(E_1|E_2)=P(E_1)$. The two most common mistakes made when calculating probabilities are 1) calculating a conditional Pr with the wrong condition and 2) assuming two events are independent when they are not. Whenever you multiply two probabilities, ask yourself if the assumption of independence is justified.

Examples 1.19

A. The probability that the first and second children of the mating *Aa* x *Aa* are *AA* and *Aa*, respectively, is given by P(*AA,Aa*) = P(*AA*)P(*Aa*) = (1/4)(1/2). The assumption of independence made here is clearly justified.

B. Consider the following more subtle example: The mating is now *A_* x *Aa*, that is, we do not know the genotype of the first parent, only the phenotype. Now, regarding the two children, P(*AA,Aa*) is not necessarily equal to P(*AA*)P(*Aa*). However, we can always write P(*AA,Aa*)= P(*AA*)P(*Aa*|*AA*). The reason the two children are no longer independent is because knowing the genotype of one of them tells us something about the genotype of the first parent which, thus, affects what we know about the other child.

C. What is the probability that a random RNA molecule of length 10 bases has at least one U? Assume A,C,G, and U are equally likely and different sites are independent. Answer: 1 - $(3/4)^{10}$

1.3.7. *Partitioning an event.*

Suppose E_1, E_2, ..., E_n are mutually exclusive and exhaustive (*i.e.*, all intersections are empty and the sum of the probabilities of the *n* events equals one). Then for any event, E, we can write

$$P(E) = \Sigma P(EE_i) = \Sigma P(E_i)P(E|E_i)$$

where the sum is over *i*=1, 2, ..., *n*.

Example 1.20

Let A = {x|x is male} and B = {x|x is over 50 years old}. Clearly A = AB or AB^c and the events "AB" and "AB^c" are mutually exclusive. (Again, draw a Venn diagram, if this is not clear to you.) Hence P(A) = P(AB) + P(AB^c). We have simply partitioned males into those over 50 and those $\leq$ 50.

1.3.8. Bayes' theorem.

From **1.3.5** and **1.3.7**, we see immediately that

$$P(E_i|E) = \frac{P(E_i)P(E|E_i)}{\sum P(E_i)P(E|E_i)}$$

This relation is called Bayes' Theorem after the Reverend Thomas Bayes, who first proposed it. Here $P(E_i)$ is referred to as the **prior probability** of E_i. $P(E_i|E)$ is the **posterior probability** of E_i. $P(E|E_i)$ is called the **likelihood**.

Examples 1.21

A. Suppose you are at a party. One of your friends comes up to you and tells you that she has discovered a 95% accurate test for a certain kind of rare liver cancer (population frequency of 1 per million). The test, if it works, would be an important aid to early diagnosis. You are impressed. However, you start to think about her claim and ask, "What do you mean when you say your test is 95% accurate?" She responds immediately, "I mean that if you have the cancer, the test will be positive 95% of the time, and if you do not have the cancer, the test will be negative 95% of the time. She goes on describing the test and finally asks, "Would you like to come to my lab and take the test?" You see no harm and agree. The next day you have your blood drawn and the test is performed. That evening your friend calls to tell you the bad news; your test was positive. Your mind suddenly clears, and you realize there is a question, the answer to which now seems very important to you: Given that I have come up positive on this test, what is the probability that I have liver cancer?

What do you know? You have four items of data.

$P(C) = 0.000001$, the frequency of this cancer is one in a million,

$P(+ \mid C) = 0.95$, if you have the cancer, the test will say so 95% of the time,

$P(- \mid \text{notC}) = 0.95$, if you are healthy, the test will say so 95% of the time,

You came up positive.

What do you want to know?

Clearly, $P(C \mid +) = ?$, What is the Pr that you have the cancer given you are positive? This is exactly the kind of question that Bayes' theorem answers.

We have
$$P(C \mid +) = \frac{P(C)P(+\mid C)}{P(C)P(+\mid C) + P(\text{notC})P(+\mid \text{notC})}$$

$$= \frac{10^{-6} \times 0.95}{10^{-6} \times 0.95 + (1-10^{-6}) \times 0.05}$$

$$= 0.000019$$

B. Suppose a woman with an albino brother and normal parents marries an albino man. Her first child is normal. What is the Pr that her second child will also be normal? Let A = "mother is heterozygote" and B = "first child is normal". Then we have

$$P(A \mid B) = \frac{P(A)P(B \mid A)}{P(A)P(B \mid A) + P(A^c)P(B \mid A^c)}$$

$$P(A^c \mid B) = \frac{P(A^c)P(B \mid A^c)}{P(A)P(B \mid A) + P(A^c)P(B \mid A^c)}$$

Thus the probability that the mother is *Aa* given that she has had one normal child is

$$\frac{(2/3)(1/2)}{(2/3)(1/2) + (1/3)(1)} = 1/2$$

Hence the risk to her next child is $(1/2)(1/2) = 1/4$.

The application of Bayes' theorem is important for understanding diagnostic or biomarker testing, as described in Example 1.21.A. However, the terminology used in those settings differs from that in our discussion above. Using the notation in the example, $P(C)$ is the *prevalence* of the disease (the prior probability). The *sensitivity* of the diagnostic test is $P(+|C)$, and its *specificity* is $P(-|notC)$. We can use Bayes' theorem and the prevalence, sensitivity, and specificity to estimate the *positive predictive value* (PPV) as $P(C|+)$ and the *negative predictive value* $P(notC|-)$.

In Example 1.21.B, you will notice that the crux of Bayes' theorem is simply that $P(E_i|E)$ is proportional to $P(E_i)P(E|E_i)$. Consequently, we can conveniently work in odds by ignoring denominators until the end. We will often use the following format in setting up problems utilizing Bayes' theorem:

Event	E_1	E_2	...	E_n
prior Pr	$P(E_1)$	$P(E_2)$	...	$P(E_n)$
likelihood	$P(E|E_1)$	$P(E|E_2)$	...	$P(E|E_n)$
posterior odds	$P(E_1)P(E|E_1)$	$P(E_2)P(E|E_2)$	...	$P(E_n)P(E|E_n)$

We may now get the posterior probabilities of $E_1 \ldots E_n$ simply by dividing each of the quantities in the "posterior odds" row by their total. In our previous example the calculations would look like this:

Event	Mother *Aa*	Mother *AA*
prior Pr	2/3	1/3
likelihood	1/2	1
posterior odds	1/3	1/3

By *prior Pr*, here, we mean the probability that the mother is a heterozygote before we know that her child is normal, that is, prior to any knowledge about the child. The *likelihood* is the probability of having a normal child if the mother is *Aa* (or *AA*). The *posterior odds* are then proportional to the product of the prior probability and the likelihood. The *posterior probability* that the mother is *Aa* is then $1/3 \div 2/3 = 1/2$.

1.4. Sample Problems

1. The first philosopher states: "Either women are wise or all men are fools." The second philosopher replies: "I deny that women are fools and men are wise." Are these two philosophers agreeing or disagreeing with each other? Hint: Use DeMorgan's rules.

2. Two committees were asked to look into the possible mishandling of a genetic counseling case by three counselors, A, B and C. The first committee concluded: "Either A and B were correct or A was correct and C was wrong." The second committee concluded "Either A was wrong or, on the other hand, B was wrong and C was right." Can both committees be correct in their findings?

3. In a recent court case, a man accused a woman of having his child and asked the court to grant him custody of the infant. The woman denied that the child is his. The man, woman and child were tested using several genetic systems. What are all the conclusions that the court could reach regarding this case? Hint: There are five.

4. Five pregnant women, each over 40 years of age, have been advised by their physicians to have amniocentesis performed. Each woman must decide first whether to have the procedure, and then if the procedure is performed and the fetus is abnormal, whether to abort or not. How many sets of decisions are possible?

5. In the pedigree below for X-linked hemophilia in which a woman, X, has two affected brothers and an unaffected son, what is the probability that X is a carrier? Use Bayes' theorem.

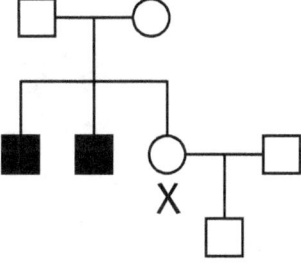

6. A sibship of size 3 consists of 1 *MM*, 1 *MN*, and 1 *NN* child. How many birth orders are possible?

7. A sibship of size 6 consists of 2 *AA*, 3 *Aa*, and 1 *aa*. How many birth orders are possible? Is this question completely unambiguous?

8. From the mating *Aa* × *Aa*, what is the Pr that the first child will either be *A_* or a heterozygote? Does rule 1.3.2 apply here?

9. Consider three autosomal loci, each with two alleles: (*A,a*), (*B,b*), (*C,c*). In a certain population, the frequencies of the eight possible gametes are: *ABC* 0.05, *ABc* 0.10, *AbC* 0.05, *Abc* 0.30, *aBC* 0.10, *aBc* 0.05, *abC* 0.10 and *abc* 0.25. We pick a gamete at random. If it contains an *A* allele, we say the event "A" has occurred, if it contains *b* and *C*, we say the event "bC" has occurred, and so on.

    a. Are the events "A" and "B" independent in this population?
    b. Are "B" and "c" independent?
    c. What is P(A|B)?
    d. What is P(Ac|B)?
    e. What is P(C|ab)?
    f. Are the events "a|B" and "C|B" independent?

10. From the mating *MN AB* × *MM OO*, what is the Pr that the first child is either *MN* or *AO* or *MMBO*?

11. Here is a challenging but useful set of problems to test your understanding of the Hardy-Weinberg rule. The diagram below depicts the sample space generated by choosing two parents and a child at random from a population in Hardy-Weinberg equilibrium for a locus with two alleles, *M* and *N*, with frequencies, *p* and *q*, respectively. There are 27 "conceivable" genotype triples (some have probability zero).

The $3 \times 3 \times 3$ conceivable families with one child when each member is classified as *MM*, *MN* or *NN*. Assume random mating.

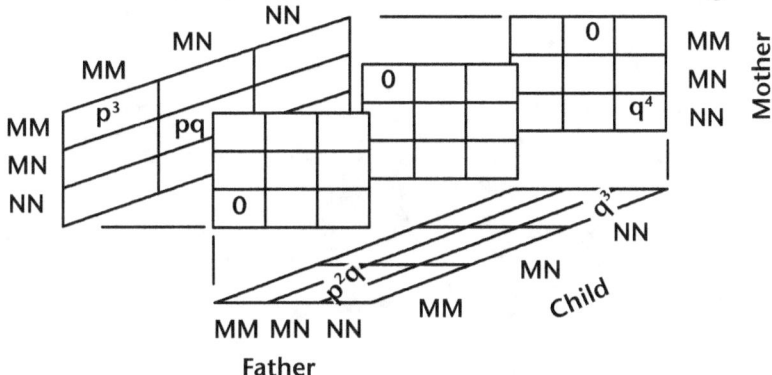

a. Fill in the cells of the diagram including marginals (some have been filled in to get you started). Letting m=mother, f=father, c=child.
b. What is the Pr that f is *MM*, m is *MM* and c is *MM*?
c. What is the Pr that f is *MN*, m is *MN* and c is N*N*?
d. What is the Pr that c is *NN* given that f is *MN* and m is *MN*?
e. What is the Pr that f is *MN* given that m is *MN* and c is *NN*?
f. Calculate Pr[f is *MN* and m is *MN* | c is *NN*).
g. Calculate Pr[f = *MN*, m=*MN* | c = *MM* or *MN*).
h. Calculate Pr[f=*MM* | m=*MN*, c=*MN*).
i. Calculate Pr[f=*MM* | m=*MM*, c=*NN*).

12. How many RNA chains of length *n* are there with exactly two U's?

13. A polypeptide of 20 amino acids has 5 histidines, 6 arginines, 4 glycines, 1 asparagine, 3 lysines, and 1 glutamic acid. How many such chains are there? What is your answer if you are told the polypeptide begins with a histidine and ends with an arginine?

2. Random Variables & Probability Distributions

In the previous chapter, we described probability as a numerical measure of chance and focused on methods for combining the probabilities of simple events. Recall that the events are considered as points in a sample space consisting of all possible events and that each event in the sample space has associated with it a measurable probability.

Probability distributions provide a kind of shorthand for describing the sample space for an experiment and its associated probabilities. In many cases, the probability distribution for an experiment can be summarized as a mathematical function. We can then use this function to calculate the probability of any particular event (or class of events) in a straightforward manner. In this chapter, we'll discuss the properties of a number of important probability distributions and their use in analyzing biological experiments.

2.1. Some Definitions

2.1.1. Distributions.

A probability distribution is a list of the events that may occur in an experiment together with their frequency or probability of occurrence. We must recognize two kinds of distributions.

a) First, the *empirical* or *sample distribution* of a specific experiment: The frequencies of the different events as they actually occurred in the experiment.

b) Second, the *population* or *theoretical distribution*: The expected frequencies with which the events would occur were we to perform an infinite number of experiments, or sampled the entire population.

Example 2.1

You have sequenced a stretch of DNA isolated from a particular organism and find that it contains a sizable open reading frame. For each of the 61 possible non-termination codons you count the number of times that the codons occur

> within the suspected orf to give the sample distribution for codon usage within this region. You may want to compare this sample distribution to the population distribution for codon usage obtained from the sequences for (ideally) all protein encoding regions or (realistically) all of the sequenced genes for the organism.

Most of the hypotheses we will want to test involve comparing two sample distributions or comparing a sample distribution to a (theoretical) population distribution.

2.1.2. Random variable.

When an event can be described numerically, for example, by counting or as a physical measurement, that event is represented by a *random variable*. We will denote the probability distribution of a random variable, x, as $f(x)$. A random variable that can take on values from a finite or countably infinite (*e.g.*, the non-negative integers) set is said to be *discrete* and its associated probability distribution is a discrete distribution. When the allowed values for the random variable are represented by an interval of real numbers, the random variable is *continuous*.

2.2. Properties of Probability Distributions

A discrete random variable, x, occurs with probability $f(x)$ and is an element of the finite or countably infinite set of all possible events X. The list of ordered pairs $(x, f(x))$ for all $x \in$ X defines the probability distribution for x. In many cases, this probability distribution may be stated as a simple mathematical formula in terms of particular parameters that specify the properties of the distribution.

A continuous random variable is defined for some interval on the line of real numbers, but the probability that a continuous random variable, x, takes on any specified real value in the interval is equal to zero. However, we can define the probability that an observation lies in a sub-interval. In particular, the cumulative distribution function, $F(x)$, is simply the probability that an observation has a value less than or equal to x. The probability density function, $f(x)$, is the derivative of the cumulative distribution function

$$f(x) = dF(x) / dx$$

or

$$F(x) = \int_{-\infty}^{x} f(u)\,du$$

2.2.1. Convergence.

The total probability in the sample space X is equal to 1, *i.e.*,

$$\sum_{x} f(x) = 1 \text{ for a discrete distribution, or}$$

$$\int_{-\infty}^{\infty} f(x)\,dx = 1 \text{ for a continuous distribution.}$$

2.2.2. Measures of location.

Several measures are used to define the location of a sample or population distribution. The most commonly used measure is the expected or mean value. This measure is defined as the sum (or integral) over all possible values of the product of the random variable and its frequency.

$$E(x) = \mu = \sum_{x} x \cdot f(x)$$

$$E(x) = \mu = \int_{-\infty}^{\infty} x \cdot f(x)\,dx$$

Another measure, the median, x_m, is defined as the value that divides the total frequency into equal halves, *i.e.*,

$$\int_{-\infty}^{x_m} f(x)\,dx = \int_{x_m}^{\infty} f(x)\,dx$$

or a similar equality involving sums for a discrete random variable. This definition is imprecise for a discrete distribution. If there are $2N+1$ members of the sample (ordered by increasing value), the median is the value of the x_{N+1} member. If there are $2N$ members, it is the value $(x_N + x_{N+1})/2$.

Similarly, quantiles (*n*-tiles) are defined as the values that divide the distribution into *n* portions containing equal (1/*n*) frequencies. For example, the second decile is the value for which 20% of the population is smaller in magnitude and the fifth decile is identical to the median.

2.2.3. Measures of dispersion.

One way to describe the dispersion, or degree of spread, in a sample distribution is to note its range, the difference between the largest and smallest observed values. However, this measure has the disadvantages of depending on only two of the observations and of tending to become larger as more observations are made. A better approach is to use the difference between two quantiles spaced on either side of the median. For example, the difference between the third and first quartiles is a range of values that contains the central half of the observations.

The most common measure of dispersion for a population is the variance, which is the average squared deviation from the mean (μ), the second equation providing a convenient formula for computation.

$$V(x) = E((x-\mu)^2) = \frac{\sum (x-\mu)^2}{n}$$

$$= E(x^2) - \mu^2 = \frac{\sum x^2}{n} - \left(\frac{\sum x}{n}\right)^2$$

For a continuous distribution, the corresponding equations are

$$V(x) = \int_{-\infty}^{\infty} (x-\mu)^2 \, f(x) dx$$

$$= E(x^2) - \mu^2 = \int x^2 \, f(x) dx - \left(\int x f(x) dx\right)^2$$

Generally, when you present your data, you would report the standard deviation (the square root of the variance) to place it in the same units as your measurements.

The above should be modified slightly in the case of a sample distribution (where you only have a subset of values drawn from a real or hypothetical population). For a sample, the variance of the sample gives a biased estimate (see Chapter 3) of the population variance, slightly underestimating it. An unbiased estimate for the population variance can be obtained by multiplying the result of the above formula by $n/(n-1)$. [It may also be noted that, while the sample variance computed in this way is unbiased, taking its square root (to obtain the standard deviation) reintroduces a bias. The magnitude of this bias is small (less than 1% for $n>30$) and routinely ignored. See Sokal and Rohlf (1995) for further details.]

Example 2.2

You have treated young mice from a sensitive inbred strain with a carcinogen. At 8 months of age, the animals were found to contain the following numbers of induced lung tumors:
47 29 23 17 25 12 13 14 16 7 12 18 29 19 30 21 19 20 17 0 24 3 9 0 10 10 18 33 26 31

Descriptive statistics for this sample are given below.

Number of observations	30
Median	18
First quartile	12
Third quartile	24.5
Mean	18.4
Standard deviation	10.4

2.3. Common Distributions in Biology

A few simple distributions provide reasonable models for a variety of biological experiments.

2.3.1. Binomial distribution.

Consider an experiment that involves some fixed number of independent trials. Each trial has two possible outcomes, conveniently termed success and failure, and the probability of success is a fixed value. We want to know the probability that x of the N trials are successes ($0 \leq x \leq N$).

Example 2.3

You know the frequency of a dominant gene, A, in a population is equal to 0.1. If you draw 5 members of the population at random, what is the probability that 3 of them will display the dominant phenotype? We assume that the population is sufficiently large that removing 5 individuals is without effect.

If the gene frequency is 0.1 (and the population is in Hardy-Weinberg equilibrium), the probability that an individual is genotype $A\_$ is equal to 0.19. Suppose that the outcome of the experiment is

Outcome = S F S S F

where S denotes an individual of genotype $A\_$. Since the trials are independent we can obtain the probability for this outcome by multiplying the probabilities of the individual events

P(Outcome)= $0.19 \times 0.81 \times 0.19 \times 0.19 \times 0.81$

$= 0.19^3 \times 0.81^2$

What we really want is the probability of obtaining 3 successes irrespective of order

$$p(A\_=3)=\binom{5}{3} \times 0.19^3 \times 0.81^2 = 0.045$$

$$\text{where } \binom{5}{3} \text{ is } 5! / (3!\, 2!)$$

The generalization of the above example is the binomial distribution. A fixed number, N, of independent trials are conducted, each of which may have one of two possible outcomes (*e.g.*, success or failure) that occur with fixed probability (*e.g.*, *p* for success and $q = (1-p)$ for failure). The probability of observing exactly *x* successes is given by

$$f(x) = \binom{N}{x} p^x q^{N-x}$$

$$x = 0, 1, 2, \ldots, N$$

$$\binom{N}{x} = N! / (x! (N-x)!)$$

The expected value and variance of the binomial distribution are

$$E(x) = Np$$

$$V(x) = Npq$$

2.3.2. Poisson distribution.

The formal derivation of the Poisson distribution concerns events that occur with constant density in time or space (an example is radioactive decay). In biological experiments this distribution commonly arises as an approximation to the binomial distribution where the number of trials, *N*, is very large and the success probability, *p*, is very small. Consider the binomial distribution where $p \ll 1$ and $N \gg x$; thus,

$$N-x+1 \approx N \text{ and}$$

$$N! / (N-x)! = N \cdot (N-1) \cdot (N-2) \ldots (N-x+1)$$

$$\approx N^x$$

You can show by expansion that

$$(1-p)^{N-x} \approx e^{-pN}$$

Substituting in the formula for the binomial distribution we obtain

$$f(x) \approx \left(\frac{N^x}{x!} \right) p^x e^{-pN}$$

remembering that *pN* is simply E(*x*), which we'll denote *m* (for mean), we obtain the Poisson distribution

$$f(x) = \frac{m^x e^{-m}}{x!} \qquad x = 0, 1, 2, \ldots$$

The mean and variance of the Poisson distribution are equal to *m*:

$$E(x) = m$$

$$V(x) = m$$

Example 2.4

You transfect a plasmid containing a selectable marker into a population of 4.5×10^5 cells and expect the plasmid to be functionally integrated into the genome with a frequency of 10^{-5}. What is the probability that you will get at least two resistant colonies?

In this case, the expected number of colonies, m, is $10^{-5}(4.5 \times 10^5)$, or 4.5. Using the Poisson distribution, we can calculate the probabilities of obtaining 0 or 1 colony

$$f(0) = (4.5^0 \, e^{-4.5}) / 0! = 0.0111$$

$$f(1) = (4.5^1 \, e^{-4.5}) / 1! = 0.0500$$

Thus,

$$P(x \geq 2) = 1 - f(0) - f(1)$$

$$= 0.939$$

2.3.3. Uniform distribution.

The discrete uniform distribution applies when all of the events in the sample space occur with equal probability. This simple distribution is useful because we can frequently transform data obtained from complex experiments so that it conforms to this distribution. This ability will be useful for hypothesis testing.

If the random variable takes on n possible values (conveniently 1 to n)

$$f(x) = 1 / n \qquad\qquad x=1,2,...,n$$

$$E(x) = (n+1) / 2$$

$$V(x) = (n+1)(n-1) / 12$$

(The expression for the variance is not intuitively obvious. If you are daring and good at algebra, you might try deriving it.)

2.3.4. Negative binomial distribution.

An interesting variation on the binomial distribution is to consider a sequence of Bernoulli trials in which N is not fixed, but is the number of trials required to obtain r "successes". In that case, the last trial must be a success, so the probability that N trials will be required to obtain r successes is given by

$$f(N) = \binom{N-1}{r-1} q^{N-r} p^{r-1} p = \binom{N-1}{r-1} p^r q^{N-r}$$

which is defined for $N \geq 1$ and $r \geq 1$, and $N \geq r$. We can rewrite this distribution by defining $s = N - r$ (taking into account that we must always perform at least r trials),

$$f(s) = \binom{r+s-1}{r-1} p^r q^s$$

In this form $E(s) = rq/p$ and $V(s) = rq/p^2$.

Example 2.5

You mate heterozygous animals to obtain a population containing mutant homozygotes that display an interesting behavioral phenotype. You want two mutants to study in detail. Because the apparatus you use to measure this phenotype can only accommodate a single animal, you test animals sequentially from the litter. What is the probability that you will obtain at least two mutants in no more than four chosen progeny?

$$f(2)=\binom{2+2-1}{2-1}\ 0.25^2\ 0.75^2=0.105$$

$$f(1)=0.094$$

$$f(0)=0.062$$

Thus, the probability that you will have at least 2 mutants in the first 4 tested animals is 0.261.

In section 2.4.3, we'll revisit the negative binomial distribution as a mixture of Poisson distributions.

2.3.5. Hypergeometric distribution.

A condition of the binomial distribution (section 2.3.1) is that the success probability, p, is invariant from one trial to the next. This condition can only be met if the trials are independent, *i.e.*, each trial is a sample taken from an infinite population (or a finite population to which we add back each item after choosing it). If instead our sample is taken from a finite population without replacement, the success probability for a particular trial depends on the outcomes of the preceding trials. For a population of size N, in which the proportion of "successes" is p ($q=1-p$), the probability of exactly x successes in k trials is given by the hypergeometric distribution

$$f(x)=\frac{\binom{pN}{x}\binom{qN}{k-x}}{\binom{N}{k}}$$

The mean and variance of the hypergeometric distribution are kp and $kpq(N-k)/(N-1)$, respectively. For k small relative to the population size N, the frequencies approach those given by the binomial distribution.

Example 2.6

You are studying a mutant mouse that you suspect will exhibit a longer lifespan than wild-type animals. You collect a group of 35 animals, of which 15 are mutant and 20 wild-type, and allow them to age. Of the last 10 animals to expire, 8 are mutant. What is the probability that 8 (or more) of the last 10 mice to die will be mutant if deaths occur at random in the population as a whole?

In this example, we "choose" a sample of 10 (k) from a population of 35 (N) animals and the probability that an animal is mutant (p) is 15/35. Thus, the probability that exactly 8 of the mice are mutant is

$$f(8) = \frac{\binom{15}{8}\binom{20}{2}}{\binom{35}{10}}$$
$$= 0.0067$$

Similarly, $f(9)$ and $f(10)$ are 5.4×10^{-4} and 1.6×10^{-5}, respectively. The probability that 8 or more mutants among the last 10 animals to die is 0.0072.

2.3.6. Normal distribution.

The normal, or Gaussian, distribution is widely applicable as a probability model for continuous random variables that may be thought of as resulting from the sum of a large number of small effects. Although the formal derivation of this distribution follows from a small number of simple assumptions, it is mathematically somewhat abstruse. More useful for our purposes, it can also be derived as an approximation to the discrete distributions we have already discussed when the number of observations is fairly large.

The normal probability density function is given by

$$f(x) = \frac{1}{\sqrt{2\pi\sigma^2}} e^{-(x-\mu)^2/2\sigma^2}$$

$$E(x) = \mu$$

$$V(x) = \sigma^2$$

Thus, the two parameters for this distribution, μ and σ^2, are the mean and variance for the distribution. The cumulative distribution is difficult to compute; most statistics books have tables (see Appendix 2) of the cumulative normal distribution standardized to

$$z = (x - \mu)/\sigma$$

such that

$$F(z) = \int_{-\infty}^{z} f(u)du = \int_{-\infty}^{z} \frac{1}{\sqrt{2\pi}} e^{-u^2/2} du$$

The utility of this distribution is a consequence of the central limit theorem. Briefly stated, this theorem demonstrates that the distribution of the sum of n independent random variables converges to a normal distribution as n becomes large. Because of this property, we will make extensive use of the normal distribution as an approximation to the distributions for test statistics that we will discuss later.

The normal distribution can also be used to approximate the distributions we discussed above. We can consider the binomial distribution in this light if we note that x, the number of successes, may be thought of as the sum of N (the number of trials) random variables, each of which may be a 0 (failure) or a 1 (success). A similar rationalization of the Poisson distribution allows us to use the central limit theorem to approximate it.

Example 2.7

What is the probability of 16 or more successes in 50 trials when the probability of success is 0.25? Using the binomial distribution, we can calculate $p(x \geq 16) = 0.1631$. Since the mean and variance for a binomial distribution are

$$E(x) = Np$$
$$V(x) = Npq$$

we calculate that the mean and standard deviation for this example are 12.5 and 3.061, respectively. The value z for the standardized normal distribution is

$$z = (16-12.5)/3.061$$
$$= 1.143$$

From a table of the standardized normal distribution
$$p(z) = 1 - F(z)$$
$$= 1 - 0.8735$$
$$= 0.1265$$

We can obtain a better approximation to a discrete distribution by applying a continuity correction. This correction takes into account the stepped shape of a discrete probability function when plotted on a real line. The correction is performed by *subtracting* 0.5 from the lower bound and *adding* 0.5 to the upper bound for the desired interval. That is, if P_D represents the probability calculated from the discrete probability distribution, m is the mean for the distribution, s is the standard deviation for that distribution, and P_N represents the probability approximated from the normal distribution

$$P_D(a \leq x \leq b) = \sum_{x=a}^{b} f(x)$$
$$\approx P_N[((a-0.5-m)/s) \leq z \leq ((b+0.5-m)/s)]$$

For the above example, we would use the corrected z value

$$z = (16-0.5-12.5)/3.061 = 0.9797$$

and from the normal table we find that $P(z \leq 0.9797) = 0.1635$, which is a closer approximation to the true probability of 0.1631. In general, the normal approximation to the binomial distribution is quite good as long as the value of p is not too close to 0 or 1 and N is moderately large (greater than 10).

2.3.7. Chi-square distribution.

A final continuous distribution that we will use extensively is the Chi-square, or χ^2, distribution, which is closely associated with the normal distribution. The distribution function for Chi-square is given by

$$F(x) = \int_0^x \frac{y^{(k/2)-1} e^{-y/2}}{2^{k/2} \Gamma(k/2)} dy$$

and is defined for $x \geq 0$. The parameter k is referred to as the number of degrees of freedom. We won't use the formula above; extensive tables of the Chi-square distribution for various values of k are provided in most statistics books (see Appendix 3). The mean and variance for the distribution are k and $2k$, respectively.

The utility of this distribution in statistics stems from two theorems (which we will not prove here). First, if we have k independent random variables that follow the standard normal distribution, then the sum of the squares of those random variables follows a Chi-square distribution with k degrees of freedom. That is, for a set of x_i ($i=1 \ldots k$) independent and identically distributed normal ($\mu=0$, $\sigma=1$) random variables, the sum

$$X = \sum_{i=1}^{k} x_i^2$$

has a Chi-square distribution with k degrees of freedom.

Another important feature of this distribution is its reproductive property; the sum of Chi-square random variables also follows a Chi-square distribution. If the k random variables X_i are independent and follow Chi-square distributions with n_i degrees of freedom, then

$$X = \sum_{i=1}^{k} X_i^2$$

follows a Chi-square distribution with $n = \sum_{i=1}^{k} n_i$ degrees of freedom.

2.4. Extensions

More often than not, biological experiments fail to conform to the simple probability models described above. We can consider a few extensions or variations on these simple univariate distributions that can take into account some of this biological variability.

2.4.1. Truncation.

It is not always possible to observe a random variable over its entire range. For example, it may not be possible to observe 0 successes in a binomial experiment, *i.e.*, the data are truncated at 1. We can evaluate the probability of a specified value for an experiment where truncation is present by dividing the probability for the value from the nontruncated distribution by the total probability for the observable values. In the above example,

$$f_t(x) = f(x) \Big/ \left\{ \sum_{x=1}^{N} f(x) \right\}$$

where $f_t(x)$ is the probability in the case of truncation and $f(x)$ is the probability for the non-truncated distribution.

Example 2.8

You are studying the frequency of spontaneous mutations at a marker locus, *a*, in T cells *in vivo*. You cross *AA* × *Aa* animals, isolate T cells from the progeny, and plate 1.5×10^5 cells to select for *aa* mutants. Note that only half of the progeny (*Aa*) can give rise to selectable mutants (assume that it is costly to simply genotype the progeny). Thus, the cultures with 0 mutants aren't really informative. If the mean mutant frequency (among cells from *Aa* animals) is 1×10^{-5}, what is the probability of obtaining 2 or fewer mutants among the samples that yielded *any* mutants?

We can use a truncated Poisson distribution (with no 0 class) to calculate this frequency. The mean number of mutants in cultures from *Aa* animals is 1.5. Thus,

---

$$f(1) = \frac{e^{-1.5} \times 1.5 / 1!}{1 - e^{-1.5}} = 0.43$$

$$f(2) = \frac{e^{-1.5} \times 1.5^2 / 2!}{1 - e^{-1.5}} = 0.32$$

The chance of obtaining 2 or fewer mutants (given that any were seen) is 0.75.

2.4.2. Multivariate distributions.

For some experiments, measurements are taken on more than one property of the system. In that case, a multivariate or joint probability distribution is required for the k variates $x_1, x_2, ..., x_k$. The multivariate extension of the binomial, the multinomial distribution, is obtained when the trials have k possible outcomes, with probabilities of occurrence $p_1 ... p_k$. The probability for a particular set of observations $x_1 ... x_k$ in N trials is

$$P(x_1, x_2, ..., x_k) = \frac{N!}{x_1! \, x_2! \, ... x_k!} \, p_1^{x_1} p_2^{x_2} \cdots p_k^{x_k}$$

where $\sum_{i=1}^{k} p_i = 1$ and $\sum_{i=1}^{k} x_i = N$

$$E(x_i) = Np_i$$
$$V(x_i) = Np_i(1 - p_i)$$
$$Cov(x_i x_j) = -Np_i p_j \qquad \text{(covariance)}$$

In the first example given in this chapter, we considered the distribution of codons in a possible open reading frame without regard to the amino acids that might be encoded. A better way to think about this problem would be to look at the distribution of codons used for particular amino acids. For example, we could consider the number of times each of the 6 possible codons for leucine were used given that there are N leucine codons in the orf as a multinomial distribution where we might take the values of the p_i from the data for all known protein encoding sequences for the organism.

Example 2.9

In a cross *Aa* × *Aa*, what is the probability of obtaining 2 *aa*,
6 *Aa*, and 4 *AA* offspring without regard to order?

The probability that an individual animal has each genotype
is 0.25, 0.5, and 0.25, respectively. The desired probability is

$$f(2,6,4) = \frac{12!}{2! \ 6! \ 4!} \ 0.25^2 \ 0.5^6 \ 0.25^4 = 0.053$$

2.4.3. Mixtures of distributions.

Even when a biological phenomenon might be expected to follow
a simple distribution, heterogeneity in one of the parameters of the parent
distribution might cause the data to fail to fit the expected distribution.
An example is the distribution of the number of tumors per animal at a
particular site in a carcinogenesis experiment. Since the process of tumor
development is a rare event occurring among a large number of target
cells at risk, we might expect these data to follow a Poisson distribution.
In fact, because of variability from animal to animal in responsiveness
(particularly for outbred animals), the number of tumors per animal generally deviates quite markedly from a Poisson distribution. In this case,
the Poisson parameter, m, varies from animal to animal. If m follows a
gamma distribution (a continuous unimodal distribution with a fat tail),
the number of tumors per mouse is described well by a negative binomial
distribution (where r is allowed to be non-integral) (Drinkwater and Klotz,
1981). The formula for the negative binomial distribution in this case differs from that shown in Section 2.3.4.

$$f(t) = \left(\frac{k}{m+k} \right)^k \frac{\Gamma(k+1)}{t! \Gamma(k)} \left(\frac{m}{m+k} \right)^t \qquad t = 0, 1, 2, ..., \infty$$

In the above formulation, m is the mean for the distribution and its variance is $m + (m^2/k)$.

The mixture of a Poisson distribution with a variety of distributions for m gives rise to a family of so-called contagious distributions that

have been applied to problems of the spread of infection in a population, clustering of accidents, and population growth.

In general if a random variable, x, follows a distribution with parameter t, $f(x \mid t)$, and t is a random variable with distribution $g(t)$, the probability distribution of x is given by

$$p(x) = \int f(x \mid t)\, g(t)\, dt$$

where the integration (or summation for a discrete $g(t)$) is taken over all possible values of t. Mixtures of distributions sometimes take fairly simple forms, but when this is not the case, the values of $p(x)$ may be evaluated numerically.

2.5. Sample Problems

1. In doing an experiment that yields "counting" data, where the observations, x, range in value from 0 to 8, you obtained the distribution indicated below. The value n_x is the number of times that you observed a value of x. Calculate the mean and variance, $E(x)$ and $V(x)$.

x	0	1	2	3	4	5	6	7	8
n_x	1	4	2	5	8	3	0	2	2

2. For a binomial distribution with N trials and success probability p, the mean number of successes is Np. Prove that this assertion is true.

3. The most rapid way to construct an inbred strain of animal is by continued brother-sister mating. Assuming that male and female offspring are equally likely, what is the probability that a litter of six animals would **not** provide a brother and a sister for mating? (Note that all would not be lost, you could set up another mating from the original parents to obtain another litter. In that case, what is the probability that two litters of six each would not provide a brother and a sister?)

4. You are interested in mutagenizing an organism at a particular locus. You use a protocol that you expect will give you 15 mutants per 1000 progeny based on experience studying a large number of genes. When you do the experiment and screen 1000 progeny, you find 25 mutants. Do you find this to be an unusually large number of mutants (based on your prior expectations)? Justify your answer.

5. You've been studying the function of a mutant gene in mice. The mutant allele (a) is present in a particular inbred strain Y and you want to study its effects on a different inbred background X that has allele A at that locus. You thus decide to make a congenic mouse strain. You begin by making an F_1 hybrid between the two strains to get mice with genotype aA. The congenic strain is constructed by repeated backcrossing of aA heterozygotes to strain X mice. The result of the first backcross is a mixture of aA and AA progeny. Normally, you would select an aA offspring and mate to a strain X mouse, but (unfortunately for you) the phenotype that results from this gene is not manifest until after the normal breeding age of the animals. To get around this

problem, you decide to randomly select some number N of the mixed group of offspring for mating to strain X mice. When the phenotypes of these animals becomes apparent, you identify a mouse that is aA in genotype and choose N of its offspring to repeat the process.

a. How large must the number N be in order for you to be 95% sure that at least one of the animals will be aA in genotype.

b. Are you being overconfident? If 5 generations of backcrossing are required, what is the chance that you will have lost the a allele by the end of this experiment?

6. You are doing a series of experiments that involve the introduction of recombinant DNA sequences into mammalian cells by transfection. For some of the experiments, you need to simultaneously introduce two different genes into the same cell. You suppose that, with the method you are using, the few cells that successfully "adopt" the exogenous DNA take up a large amount of DNA, such that co-introduction of two markers is a likely event. In order to test this assumption, you do the following experiment:

Cells are simultaneously transfected with equal quantities of two types of DNA that express independent selectable markers "A" and "B." After treatment, you divide the cells into two parts. For one group, you seed 6 dishes with 100 cells each and select for the presence of marker A. For the other group, you seed 6 dishes with 100 cells each and select for marker B. You observe the following numbers of colonies.

Group 1 (A⁺):   6, 11, 7, 13, 10, 9
Group 2 (B⁺):   9, 9, 10, 7, 9, 11

You now isolate 10 colonies from the group 1 (A⁺) dishes and score each cell clone for expression of the B marker. You find that 8 of the 10 colonies selected for "A" also express "B." How likely is this result (or more extreme) if your initial assumption were false, that is, A and B markers are taken up independently?

7. You believe (from the results of other experiments) that a particular protein "X" increases the expression of genes linked to a specific promoter. In order to test this hypothesis, you construct 8 matched pairs of cell lines: one member of each pair expresses "X" at a high level and

in the other, "X" is not expressed. Into each cell line, you introduce DNA in which the promoter of interest is linked to a reporter gene and measure the amount of transcription of the reporter gene by an RNA dot blot.

Cell line pair	cpm hybridization no "X"	cpm hybridization with "X"
1	300	450
2	210	85
3	900	1300
4	750	950
5	490	375
6	50	95
7	195	500
8	650	1400

Construct a test of your hypothesis. [Hint: Consider this to be a binomial experiment with 8 trials and rephrase your null hypothesis (*i.e.*, of no difference within a pair) with that in mind.]

8. We will most often use the normal approximation to a discrete distribution to compute the probability in the upper tail of a distribution, *i.e.*, for a value b, the sum of all probabilities from b to the maximum value for the distribution. It's worth knowing how good these approximations are for a given distribution.

For the Poisson distribution, compare the exact and normal approximation upper tail probabilities for values of x greater than $m + (m)^{0.5}$, $m + 2(m)^{0.5}$, and $m + 3(m)^{0.5}$ for values of m (the mean for the distribution) of 1 and 8. Round the above values of x to the nearest integer. [Note: This problem is fairly easy if you are handy with computers. If you would rather do the problem by hand, consider the following helpful hints. First, you only need to compute the exact probabilities once for a given value of m and you don't want to add up all of the exact probabilities to ∞. To save time, compute the normal approximation for $m + 3(m)^{0.5}$ first. Then start computing exact Poisson probabilities from the nearest integer to $m + (m)^{0.5}$ up to a value such that p(x) is 0.001 × the above normal approximation. Second, there is an easy way to compute successive Poisson probabilities. Note that

$$p(x + 1) = p(x) \times m \, / \, (x + 1)$$

Using the above formula will save you lots of time.]

9. Mice with the genotype *a/a +/c^{ch}* will occasionally develop light brown spots in their coats as a consequence of a somatic mutation in the wild type allele at the albino (*c*) locus that occurs during the proliferation of melanoblasts *in utero*. You've been studying a mutation in a gene (*z*) that you believe should increase the rate at which somatic mutations would occur. You do the following cross [*Z/z a/a c^{ch}/c^{ch}*] × [*Z/z a/a +/+*]. Say that you expect that the number of spots per offspring would be Poisson distributed with the mean number of spots (*m*) depending on the genotype at the *Z* locus: *Z/Z*, *m* = 0.8; *Z/z*, *m* = 2.0; *z/z*, *m* = 10. What would be the distribution of the number of spots per mouse from the above cross? Graph the distribution.

3. ESTIMATION

We will often want to use the set of observed values obtained in an experiment, that is, the sample distribution for the random variable, in order to infer, or estimate, properties of the population from which the sample was drawn. These properties might include the mean or variance of the population distribution or parameters of the distribution function (*e.g.*, the success probability for a binomial distribution). In genetics, we will often be interested in estimating such quantities as gene frequencies, recombination frequencies, or mutation rates. While most of this book focuses on nonparametric statistics, in which the form of the population distribution is not assumed to be known, it is worth discussing briefly some properties of estimators and a general method for obtaining a class of estimators with useful properties. We will also discuss the use of confidence limits to provide a measure of the quality of our estimates and describe an approach to using the sample data to obtain confidence limits for parameters when the form of the population distribution is unknown.

3.1. Properties of Estimators

The process of estimation is analogous to that of measurement. When we measure some quantity (weight, blood pressure, *etc.*) we want our result to be accurate (close to the true value) and precise (highly reproducible from measurement to measurement). The same considerations apply to problems of estimation in which we seek estimators that are unbiased and consistent. Consider a sample consisting of n observations, from which we can define an estimator, $\hat{p}$, for a parameter p. If this estimator is unbiased, then

$$E(\hat{p}) = p \text{ for all values of } n.$$

Another desirable property for estimators is consistency, *i.e.*, the estimated value should converge on the true value as the number of observations increases. In terms of probability, for any positive value of ε (however small):

$$P[|p - \hat{p}| > \varepsilon] \to 0 \quad \text{as} \quad n \to \infty$$

Given a choice of estimators that are unbiased and consistent, we would obviously prefer the one with the smallest
variance. In the figure at right, the top
panel depicts two alternative estimators.
One of the estimators, the one with the
smaller variance (narrower distribution),
is biased because the mean value is different from the true value of p. In the
bottom panel, distributions for an unbiased, consistent estimator are depicted.
Consider the following question: Which
of the two estimators shown in the upper panel (the unbiased one or the one
with the smaller variance) is likely to be
most useful to you?

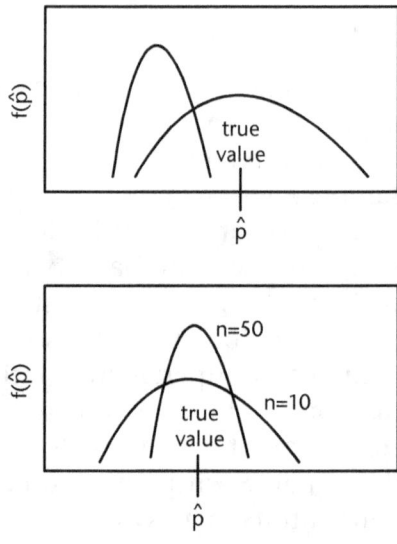

3.2. Maximum Likelihood Estimation

Consider an experiment in which we make n, independent obser-
vations of the random variable x which follow a distribution $f(x \mid \mathbf{p})$ where
$\mathbf{p}$ is the vector of parameters (*i.e.*, $\{p_1, p_2, ..., p_k\}$) for the distribution. The
probability for obtaining the particular results for this experiment, the
likelihood, is given by

$$L(x_1 x_2 ... x_n) = \prod_{i=1}^{n} f(x_i \mid \mathbf{p})$$

The above expression is simply the product of the probabilities of obtaining the observations in our experiment, given the parameters for the distribution, and follows from the previous definition of independence and
the product rule.

The use of the sample likelihood function in problems of hypothesis testing and estimation was first proposed by R. A. Fisher in 1925 (Fisher, 1973). This approach has a strong intuitive appeal. If we have two hypotheses that differ in the values of the parameters $\mathbf{p}$, it seems quite natural to favor the hypothesis that yields the higher likelihood and that the
ratio of the likelihoods would give us a measure of the confidence with
which we should prefer that hypothesis. The use of *likelihood ratio* tests for

statistical inference is an important topic because these tests have the general property of being the most powerful (see Chapter 4) for any case in which the form of the distribution function can be specified. Although we won't be able to cover this topic, the efficiencies of the statistical tests we discuss later will be considered relative to the appropriate likelihood ratio test.

We most often will be interested in testing hypotheses that do not specify precisely the values of the parameters of the distributions but only the form. What method should we then use to estimate the parameters under the hypothesis? Again, it seems natural to use an estimate that gives the highest possible likelihood under the hypothesis. This estimator, the *maximum likelihood estimator* (MLE), has, as will be discussed below, several important properties that make it the estimator of choice in a variety of experimental situations. Traditional and modern linkage analysis is, for example, dominated by the concept of likelihood and maximum likelihood estimation.

3.2.1. Determining the Maximum Likelihood Estimator.

The basic idea underlying maximum likelihood estimation is rather simple: You write down, in terms of the parameter to be estimated, the probability of what you observed, and then choose as your estimate of that parameter the value that maximizes this probability. Although the idea is straightforward, sometimes the implementation is difficult. We will stick to relatively simple examples below and describe three methods for obtaining an MLE: the analytic approach, numerical methods, and the EM algorithm. Our first example uses the analytic method to obtain the MLE for the binomial success probability, p.

Example 3.1

You want to estimate the frequency of recombination between two loci, A and B, and set up the following test cross:

$$\frac{a \quad b}{a \quad b} \times \frac{A \quad B}{a \quad b}$$

You observe the following distribution of genotypes for 30 progeny (only the haplotype from the father is shown)

Genotype	No. of Progeny
A B	13
A b	2
a B	1
a b	14

Thus, you observed 3 recombinant animals in your set of 30. Since the animals are "independent" and each is either a recombinant (success) or non-recombinant (failure), the number of observed recombinants, x, in a collection of N offspring should follow a binomial distribution with a parameter p, which is the probability of recombination.

$$f(x) = \binom{N}{x} p^x (1-p)^{N-x}$$

For the binomial distribution, we could view our experiment as N trials of one observation each. Thus, the likelihood function is

$$L = p^x (1-p)^{N-x}$$

We can obtain the maximum likelihood estimate, $\hat{p}$, of the success probability by setting the derivative of the likelihood function to 0 and solving for p.

In deriving the maximum likelihood estimator for a parameter it is often more convenient to work with the *log* of the likelihood, in order to convert the product in the likelihood function to a sum. The value of p that maximizes $\ln(L)$ will also maximize L. For our example, the *log* likelihood and its derivative are

$$\ln(L) = x \ln p + (N - x) \ln(1 - p)$$
$$\frac{d \ln(L)}{dp} = \frac{x}{p} + (N - x)\frac{(-1)}{1 - p}$$

To obtain the maximum likelihood estimator, $\hat{p}$, we can set the derivative to 0 and solve for p

$$\frac{x}{\hat{p}} = \frac{N-x}{1-\hat{p}}$$

$$\hat{p} = \frac{x}{N}$$

The above estimator should come as no surprise, since it is the one you would use quite naturally. It is often the case that, when there is an intuitively obvious estimator, it is also the maximum likelihood estimator.

Without deriving it, we'll note that the variance for the maximum likelihood estimator of p can be obtained by taking the second derivative of the likelihood function (see below). The variance is –1 times the expected value for the reciprocal of the second derivative of the log likelihood:

$$V(\hat{p})^{-1} = -E\left[\frac{d^2 \ln L}{dp^2}\right]$$

$$= E\left[\frac{x}{p^2} + \frac{N-x}{(1-p)^2}\right]$$

$$= \frac{E[x]}{p^2} + \frac{E[N-x]}{(1-p)^2}$$

$$= \frac{Np}{p^2} + \frac{N(1-p)}{(1-p)^2}$$

$$= \frac{N}{p(1-p)}$$

Thus, our variance is

$$V(\hat{p}) = \frac{p(1-p)}{N}$$

which can be estimated by substituting $\hat{p}$ for p in the right hand side of the equation.

> **Example 3.1 (continued)**
>
> For our test cross, the maximum likelihood estimate for the probability of recombination is
>
> $$\hat{p} = \frac{3}{30} = 0.10$$
>
> and its standard deviation (the square root of the variance) is estimated to be
>
> $$\sqrt{V(\hat{p})} = \left(\frac{0.1 \times 0.9}{30}\right)^{0.5} = 0.0548$$
>
> We can compute the likelihood for our experiment under the condition that the recombination probability is 0.10 from
>
> $$L = 0.1^3 \times 0.9^{27} = 5.815 \times 10^{-5}$$
>
> You can satisfy yourself that 0.1 is the maximum likelihood estimate by trying a few alternative values. For example, the likelihoods for p=0.11 and 0.09 are 5.724×10^{-5} and 5.713×10^{-5}, respectively.

A similar approach can be used to obtain estimates for multiple parameters of more complex likelihood functions. The partial derivative of the *log* likelihood with respect to each parameter is set to 0 and the resulting set of equations is solved for the parameters. In this case, the parameters will covary and we will need to invert a matrix of the partial second derivatives to determine the variances and covariances of the parameters.

3.2.2. Properties of MLEs.

If we use MLE theory, is our estimate a good one? Obviously, it depends on what we mean by *good*. Statisticians have defined various properties of *goodness* precisely. Under rather general conditions, maximum likelihood estimators (MLE) have many of these properties. Here are some of those properties; the value of most should make intuitive sense to you.

*MLEs are **consistent**.* As described in section 3.1, this assertion means that the estimator converges in probability to the true value of the parameter as the sample size increases. In other words, the more information we have, the better our estimator will be. Implicit in this discussion is a concept that is crucially important to an understanding of statistical methods: Estimators have distributions. If you sample over and over, your estimator won't yield the same estimate every time because the values in the sample will vary randomly. If you plot the estimates from a large number of samples, you want the resulting distribution of estimates to be closely concentrated around the true value of the parameter, and it would certainly be useful if the concentration became tighter for larger samples. That case is the property of consistency.

*MLEs tend to **normality** as the sample size gets large.* This property is useful because the normal distribution is nicely symmetrical and a great deal is known about it (see section 2.3.6).

*MLEs have a built in (asymptotic) **variance formula**.* For reasonably large sample sizes, the variance of an MLE is given by the formula

$$V(\hat{p}) = \frac{-1}{E(d^2 \ln L / dp^2)}$$

where *V* is the variance and *E* refers to the expectation. We might ask why the variance of the estimator would have anything to do with the second derivative of the *log* likelihood. Remember, the likelihood is a function of *p* whose graph is a unimodal curve. The first derivative of the *log* likelihood gives us the slope of the curve at any value of *p*. The second derivative tells us how fast that slope is changing with changes in *p*. If the slope is changing slowly (the second derivative is small), then the likelihood is relatively flat around the maximum. If the slope is changing quickly (the second derivative is large), the likelihood function is rather steep around the maximum. If the likelihood is rather flat, then the value of *p* corresponding to the maximum likelihood is not much more likely than nearby values of *p*. On the other hand, if the curve is steep, the maximum likelihood estimate is considerably more likely than most other values of *p*.

The second derivative, thus, is a measure of how much information we have about the unknown p. A large second derivative means lots of information (small variance), while a small second derivative means little information (large variance). Hence the obscure sounding relationship: the large sample variance of the MLE equals the reciprocal of minus the average value of the second derivative of the log of the likelihood. Large, here, is hard to define precisely. The formula is only exact at a sample size of infinity, but $N=30$ is generally close enough to infinity for us to use the formula.

*MLEs are **efficient**.* This statement means that, under rather general assumptions, MLEs have a smaller variance (more information) than other kinds of estimators, at least in large samples. In fact, they often have the smallest variance possible.

*MLEs are **sufficient**.* Sufficiency is the most important general property of MLEs, but is also the most subtle. Loosely, it means that an MLE always uses all of the *information* in the sample. However, that is not a very informative statement unless the term *information* is carefully defined. What is meant is that the distribution of the sample, given the MLE, is independent of the unknown parameter. This concept is both interesting and deep, but a simple example may make it easier to assimilate. Suppose we wish to estimate the probability, p, of observing heads by flipping a coin 100 times. We observe 40 heads (and our MLE will therefore be 0.4). Note that in deriving this estimate, we do not need to know the order in which the heads or tails were observed (there are 100!/40!60! equally likely orders). In some sense then, the proportion of heads observed embodies all of the information in the sample there is concerning the unknown parameter, p. So the observed proportion of heads is a sufficient estimator of p.

*MLEs are **invariant**.* This very useful property means that if $\hat{p}$ is the MLE of p, and f(p) is some function of p, then f($\hat{p}$) is the MLE of f(p). For example, the MLE of p^2 is $\hat{p}^2$.

*MLEs are **not**, in general, **unbiased**.* Unfortunately, it is not, in general, true that the average of the MLE equals the unknown parameter for finite sample size. Of course, even if an MLE is biased at finite sample sizes, it will become less so as the sample size gets larger because MLEs are consistent. Sometimes the exact bias is known. For example, the '*n*-1' in the formula for the sample variance is a correction for bias.

3.2.3. Numerical methods for maximum likelihood estimation.

Deriving a closed expression for a maximum likelihood estimator is not always as straightforward as it was above for the binomial distribution. In such cases we can use numerical methods to obtain the estimator by computing the *log* likelihood as a function of the parameter of interest and finding the value of the parameter that gives the highest (*i.e.*, least negative) *log* likelihood. As shown in the example below, this procedure is relatively simple to perform for distributions with a single parameter, but it can also be applied simultaneously for any arbitrary number of parameters.

Example 3.2

You have been studying a gene that causes coat color spots in mice as a consequence of somatic mutation in pigment cells and you are interested in the effect of the genetic background of the animals on the frequency of these somatic mutations. Animals heterozygous for this gene (*D* / +) develop the spots, but the homozygous mutant mice die before birth. You mate heterozygous mutant mice with wild type animals from a different strain and analyze the progeny for the number of spots. Since these somatic mutations are presumably rare events, you imagine that the number of spots per mutant animal should follow a Poisson distribution and you wish to estimate the Poisson parameter, *m*, for a variety of matings of mutant mice to different strains. Note that only half of the offspring will carry the mutant gene so that the "zero" class, the animals with no spots will contain both irrelevant mice (+/+) and *D*/+ mice that develop no spots. Thus, the distribution of the number of spots, *x*, per mouse (among mice that contain spots) will be a truncated Poisson distribution

---

$$f(x) = \left\{\frac{e^{-m}m^x}{x!}\right\} \Big/ \left\{1 - e^{-m}\right\}$$

Among 25 animals that display spots, we observe

Number of spots (x_i)	Number of mice (n_i)
1	8
2	7
3	4
4	3
5	3

We can compute the *log* likelihood as

$$\log L = \sum_{i=1}^{5} n_i \log(f(x_i))$$

We can find the maximum likelihood estimate for *m* by using a set of trial values and zeroing in on the maximum by Newton's method. We have plotted the log likelihood function below

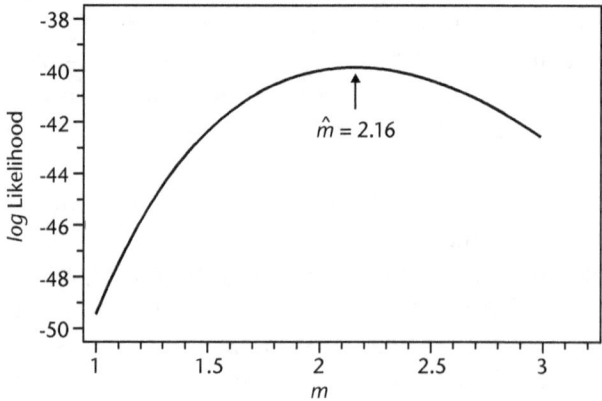

Estimating the variance of $\hat{m}$ numerically, we obtain 0.187. Thus, the MLE for *m* is 2.16 ± 0.43.

3.2.4. *The EM algorithm.*

Because of dominance and epistasis, genetic experiments often pose the problem of obtaining maximum likelihood estimates in the face of incomplete data. For example, in crosses involving two loci with dominant alleles, the presence of both recombinant and non-recombinant offspring in some phenotypic classes may make it impossible to simply count recombinants, as we did in Example 3.1, to obtain an estimate of the recombination frequency. The Expectation Maximization (EM) algorithm provides an iterative approach to obtaining maximum likelihood estimates in such cases.

In our example of linkage between dominant markers, we would apply the EM algorithm as follows.

1. We obtain (or just guess) the value of the recombination fraction, r, by some simple method.

2. We use this value of r and our observed phenotypes to calculate the expected numbers of recombinants and non-recombinants under the assumption that the estimate is correct and we can distinguish all of the genotypes.

3. We use the above expectations to obtain the MLE for r, which is simply the expected number of recombinants divided by the number of progeny.

4. Repeat steps 2 and 3 until successive estimates differ by less than some specified, small amount, giving us the MLE, $\hat{r}$.

The EM algorithm is a powerful, general method for obtaining maximum likelihood estimates and tends to converge quickly. There are also methods (too complex to provide in detail here) using this approach to obtain estimates of the variance of the estimator. In general, it is wise to try several starting values for the parameter in case the likelihood surface is multimodal.

Example 3.3

We are analyzing the results of the mating (uppercase indicating the dominant alleles)

$$\frac{A \quad B}{a \quad b} \times \frac{A \quad b}{a \quad b}$$

from which we obtain 5 offspring with the AB phenotype, 3 of Ab, 1 of aB and 1 of ab. The genotype frequencies (as a function of r) for this mating are

	Ab	ab
AB	(1-r)/4	(1-r)/4
aB	r/4	r/4
Ab	r/4	r/4
ab	(1-r)/4	(1-r)/4

The AB phenotype is comprised of three genotypes (indicated by the shading), *AB/Ab*, *AB/ab*, and *aB/Ab*, the last of which is recombinant. Among these AB offspring, the proportion of recombinants is

$$P[recomb.|AB] = \frac{r/4}{\left(\frac{1-r}{4}\right) + \frac{r}{4} + \left(\frac{1-r}{4}\right)}$$

$$= \frac{r}{2-r}$$

Thus, the expected number of recombinants in the AB phenotypic class is $5r/(2-r)$. Similarly, the expected number of recombinants for the Ab class is $3(2r)/(1+r)$. All of the aB offspring and none of the ab offspring are recombinant.

To apply the EM algorithm to obtaining the MLE of r, let's use 0.5 (*i.e.*, non-linkage) as our starting value.

The expected number of recombinants, R, given $r=0.5$ and our observed phenotypes is

$$E[R] = \frac{5 \times 0.5}{2 - 0.5} + \frac{3 \times 2 \times 0.5}{1 + 0.5} + 1$$
$$= 1.6667 + 2 + 1$$
$$= 4.6667$$

This expected value gives us a new estimate of r of 0.46667 (dividing the $E[R]$ by the number of offspring). We use this estimate to again obtain the expected number of recombinants and a new estimate of r. The complete sequence of iterations to estimate $\hat{r}$ to 5 decimal places is

0.50000 0.46667 0.44308 0.42652 0.41493 0.40684
0.40119 0.39726 0.39452 0.39261 0.39128 0.39036
0.38971 0.38926 0.38895 0.38873 0.38858 0.38847
0.38840 0.38835 0.38831 0.38829 0.38827 0.38826
0.38825 0.38824 0.38824

We converge to the same value, starting from $r=0.1$.

Our MLE, $\hat{r}$, is 0.388 (with a variance, V($\hat{r}$) of 0.072).

3.3. Confidence Limits

The variance of an estimator, obtained above from the second derivative of the likelihood function, provides a measure of its precision. Alternatively we could define a range of values for the parameter, a confidence interval, for which we can assert that the probability is greater than or equal to $1-\alpha$ that this interval contains the true value of the parameter. In the discussion above, we focused on methods to obtain a unique estimate of a parameter, $\hat{p}$, based on our set of observations. We could instead devise a new method that specifies a range of values for the parameter. If we did our experiment a large number of times, the estimated range for the parameter is a confidence interval if the range contained the true value of the parameter in $100(1-\alpha)$ percent of the trials. In the discussion below, we will describe methods for determining the confidence interval for the binomial success probability, but the same approaches can be used in any case that we can model our experiment with an easily computed distribution function. We will also discuss a powerful method for obtaining confidence limits when the form of the appropriate population distribution is unknown.

3.3.1. Binomial confidence limits.

Estimating the confidence limits for the binomial paramater, p, is straightforward, if somewhat computationally intensive. As an example, consider the linkage experiment discussed above (Example 3.1). We observed 3 recombinant animals in a sample of 30, giving us a maximum likelihood estimator for the recombination frequency equal to 0.1. We wish to compute the 95% confidence limits for this frequency. In order to obtain the upper confidence limit, we want to determine the value p_u such that the probability of obtaining 3 or fewer recombinants would be smaller than 0.025 if the true recombination frequency were equal to p_u. Using the binomial distribution we can compute for various values of p, the probability

$$P = \sum_{i=0}^{3} \binom{30}{i} p^i (1-p)^{30-i}$$

We can similarly define the lower bound for the confidence interval, p_l, as the value of p that gives a probability of 0.025 for obtaining 3 or more recombinants

$$P = \sum_{i=3}^{30} \binom{30}{i} p^i (1-p)^{30-i}$$

Setting each of the cumulative binomial probabilities above to 0.025, we need to solve for p to obtain our confidence limits. Although it is not possible to arrive at a solution algebraically, we can use numerical methods to estimate p. The simplest such approach is the bisection method for finding the root of the equation $P-0.025=0$. Choose a starting value for p and continue to alter the value until the above difference changes sign, *i.e.*, we've bracketed the interval containing the value of p. Compute the value of the function at the midpoint of the interval and replace the endpoint of the same sign to yield a new interval of half the size. Repeat this process until we have an interval of the desired small size. The table below shows the results for estimation of p_u.

Interval	p	P-0.025
	0.4	0.0247
	0.2	-0.0977
[0.2,0.4]	0.3	0.0157
[0.2,0.3]	0.25	-0.0125
[0.25,0.3]	0.275	0.0058
[0.25,0.275]	0.2625	-0.0020
[0.2625,0.275]	0.26875	0.0022
[0.2625,0.26875]	0.26562	0.0002
[0.2625,0.26562]	0.26406	-0.0008
[0.26406,0.26562]	0.26484	-0.0003
[0.26484,0.26562]	0.26523	-0.00004

Thus, we obtain an upper confidence limit of approximately 0.265. Using an analogous approach, considering the probability of obtaining 3 or more recombinants as a function of p, we obtain a lower confidence limit of 0.021. Thus, the 95% confidence interval for our estimate of the recombination frequency is (0.021, 0.265). Note carefully the meaning of this confidence interval. It is **not** appropriate to say that there is a 95% probability that the true value for the recombination fraction lies in the interval (0.021, 0.265) because the true value is fixed. We can say that, if we repeated this experiment many times and estimated the confidence interval for each replicate as we did above, 95% of these intervals would contain the true value.

Estimating the confidence interval for the binomial parameter as described above would be difficult to perform without the aid of a computer. However, we can take advantage of the normal approximation to the binomial distribution (see Example 2.7) to compute more simply an approximate confidence interval.

Recall that the mean for the binomial distribution is equal to Np, and its variance is $Np(1-p)$. We can use the standard normal distribution ($\mu=0$, $\sigma=1$) to approximate the distribution of the number of successes, x, using the transformation $z=(x-\mu)/\sigma$.

In order to define the endpoints for the $(1-\alpha)$ confidence interval, we can use the tabulated, cumulative standard normal distribution (Appendix 2) by finding the value of z that yields an upper tail probability of $\alpha/2$. For the 90%, 95%, and 99% confidence intervals, the appropriate values of z are 1.64, 1.96, and 2.57, respectively. The lower and upper confidence limits for p satisfy the equations

$$Z = \frac{x - (Np_l) - 0.5}{\sqrt{Np_l(1-p_l)}}$$

$$-Z = \frac{x - (Np_u) + 0.5}{\sqrt{Np_u(1-p_u)}}$$

Solving the above equations for p_l and p_u, we obtain

$$p_l = \frac{N(2(x-0.5)+Z^2) - \sqrt{(N(2(x-0.5)+Z^2))^2 - 4N(N+Z^2)(x-0.5)^2}}{2(N(N+Z^2))}$$

$$p_u = \frac{N(2(x+0.5)+Z^2) + \sqrt{(N(2(x+0.5)+Z^2))^2 - 4N(N+Z^2)(x+0.5)^2}}{2(N(N+Z^2))}$$

In applying these approximations, note that p_l can not be less than 0 nor p_u greater than 1. For the problem detailed in Example 3.1, we would obtain approximate 95% confidence limits for p of (0.026, 0.277), which may be compared to the interval (0.021, 0.265) we determined above by iteration. When the binomial distribution is more nearly normal, a better approximation to the confidence limits is obtained. For example, if we had observed 30 recombinants in 120 offspring, the approximate 95% confidence limits for the recombination fraction would be (0.177, 0.339), while those obtained iteratively using the binomial distribution are (0.175, 0.337).

3.3.2. Bootstrap confidence intervals.

Using the above method to determine the confidence limits for an estimator depends on our ability to specify the type of probability distribution that adequately describes the population from which our sample was taken. Unfortunately, in many experiments we will only have a dim idea of the nature of the appropriate population distribution. The bootstrap method, first discussed in detail by Efron (1979; Efron and Tibshirani, 1993), is based on the idea that, in the absence of other information, the distribution of values in our sample (the empirical distribution) is the best model for the population distribution. We can model the distribution of our estimator by repeatedly re-sampling our set of observations and computing the estimator for each new sample.

The most frequent application of the bootstrap method is to determine confidence limits for estimators, such as the mean, variance, or median. Application of this method is straightforward, though computationally intensive. Consider the problem of determining the 95% confidence limits for the mean of a set of N observations. We construct a bootstrap sample by choosing at random one of our observations and noting its value. We return that observation to the pool and repeat the process until we obtain a set of N randomly chosen values and compute the mean of our new random sample. That is, we are *sampling with replacement* from our original set of observations. If we construct 1000 bootstrap samples and determine the mean of each, we can approximate the confidence interval for our sample mean by putting our bootstrap means in increasing order and taking the 25th (*i.e.*, the 2.5 percentile point) and 975th values in the list.

Example 3.4

You are comparing the efficacies of the standard therapy for a particular type of cancer with a new treatment. Patients are assigned at random to the two treatments and you observe the length of time (in months) that each survives. The ordered survival times for the two groups are

Standard (*n*=32): 1.5 1.5 1.5 1.5 1.5 1.5 1.5 1.5 2.5 2.5 2.5 2.5 3 4.5 4.5 4.5 5 5 6 6 7 7 8 8 8 8 11 15 16 26 33

New (*n*=26): 1.5 2.5 2.5 3.5 3.5 6.5 8.5 8.5 8.5 9.5 10.5 13 13 13 13 14 14 15 15 19 21 26 26 35 35 42

The median survival times for the Standard and New therapies are 4.75 and 13 months, respectively. What are the 95% confidence limits for these medians?

Construct 10000 bootstrap samples by choosing with replacement 32 values from the set of Standard observations
and determine the median of each sample. The first few medians are

5 4.5 3 4.75 2.75 4.75 4.75 4.5 4.75 5.5 7 5 4.5 2.5 6 5.5
4.75 6 ...

Placing our 10000 medians in order, we find that the 250th
and 9750th values are 2.5 and 7, respectively. Thus, the 95%
confidence limits for the median survival on the Standard
therapy are (2.5,7).

A similar approach yields 95% confidence limits for median
survival on the new therapy of (8.5,15). Given that the confidence limits for the two treatments do not overlap, we
would have a good reason to prefer the new therapy.

Although a number of more sophisticated methods for determining the bootstrap confidence limits of an estimator have been devised,
largely to reduce bias in the case that the distribution of the data is highly
skewed, the simple approach described above has been shown to perform
well under most circumstances. A detailed discussion of various bootstrap
methods can be found in Bryan Manly's book, Randomization, Bootstrap
and Monte Carlo Methods in Biology (2001).

How many bootstrap samples are required? Based on several studies, Manly suggests at least 1000 resamplings for 95% confidence limits,
scaling upward as α decreases (e.g., 5000 trials for the 99% confidence limits). The great increase in readily available computing power over the last
decade has generated increasing interest in the bootstrap and other
"computationally intensive" methods. When first proposed by Efron in
1979, bootstrap methods required access to a mainframe computer. The
10,000 re-samplings used in the example above to generate the confidence interval for a median required less than 0.03 seconds on a mid-
range desktop computer.

3.4. Expectations and Variances of Functions

We often are interested in derived quantities obtained from measurements on one or more random variables. Examples include normalizing the number of counts in a particular band on a Southern blot to a reference band in the same lane or calculating the volume of a sphere from its measured diameter. We can broaden the definitions for expectation and variance to include any function $g(x)$ of a random variable x as follows

$$E[g(x)] = \int g(x)f(x)dx$$

$$V[g(x)] = \int \{g(x) - E[g(x)]\}^2 f(x)dx$$

where $f(x)$ is the distribution of x and the integral is taken to indicate summation for a discrete variable. Calculating these values explicitly for most distributions and functions is not easy. An approximate method is available that is generally accurate to order $1/n$ where n is the number of measurements.

For a function of a single random variable $g(x)$ where the mean of x is m and the variance of x is $V(x)$

$$E[g(x)] \approx g(m)$$

$$V[g(x)] \approx \{dg/dx\}^2 V(x)$$

where the derivative is evaluated at m.

A similar approximate method may be used for functions of several random variables using partial derivatives. For most purposes, it will suffice to consider functions of two random variables, x and y, involving constants, a and b. When working with two random variables it is useful to define their covariance

$$Cov(x,y) = E(xy) - E(x)E(y)$$

Note that if x and y are independent, the covariance is equal to 0.

The table below gives the expectation and variance for several common functions.

Function	Expectation	Variance
$ax + b$	$aE(x) + b$	$a^2 V(x)$
$x + y$	$E(x) + E(y)$	$V(x) + V(y) + 2\,\mathrm{Cov}(x,y)$
$x\,y$ (independent)	$E(x)\,E(y)$	$V(x)E^2(y) + V(y)E^2(x) + V(x)V(y)$
x/y (independent)	$E(x)/E(y)$	$\left\{\dfrac{E(x)}{E(y)}\right\}^2 \times \left\{\dfrac{V(x)}{E^2(x)} + \dfrac{V(y)}{E^2(y)}\right\}$

where $E^2(x) = \{E(x)\}^2$

Example 3.5

Extracts are prepared from cells co-transfected with an expression plasmid and with a control vector or one carrying a dominant negative mutant of a particular transcription factor. The extracts are assayed for luciferase activity, giving the following values (relative light units):

Control: 2127120, 1235417, 1053546, 1571762
Dom. Neg: 320310, 265511, 373367, 452025

What is the activity in the dominant negative transfections normalized to the control activity? The mean and variances are

E(control) = 1.497×10^6; V(control) = 2.226×10^{11}
E(mutant) = 3.528×10^5; V(mutant) = 6.314×10^9

mutant/control = 0.24 ± 0.09

3.5. An Aside on Significant Figures

In reporting your results, it is important to be mindful of the number of significant figures presented for measurements or derived quantities, such as means and standard deviations. It is fairly easy to deal with issues related to the precision of the tool that you used to obtain the measurement. You should not imply that your measurement is more precise than it was. For example, if you weighed tissues on a balance that was accurate to the nearest mg, you obviously should not represent the mean for a group of animals as 115.2357 mg.

A more subtle problem arises when experimental variability (as a consequence of randomness in the biological process you are studying) greatly exceeds the variability introduced by your measuring tool. One approach, suggested by Sokal and Rohlf (1995), is to obtain your measurements (*i.e.*, record the value to the number of significant figures) such that the number of unit steps between the smallest and largest values in the set is between 30 and 300. For example, if you are measuring bone length in a group of animals and the observations range from 1.0 to 1.3 cm, you should use a tool that will measure to an accuracy of 0.01 cm (and report means and standard deviations to that precision).

Our bias is to use the magnitude of the standard deviation as a guide and to report the data to one or two significant figures in the standard deviation and the mean value to the same decimal place. For example, in the luminometer data given in Example 3.5, the means (± standard deviation) for the control and mutant constructs would be reported as $(15 \pm 4) \times 10^5$ and $(3.5 \pm 0.7) \times 10^5$, respectively.

3.6. Sample Problems

1. For the Poisson distribution, the natural estimator for the parameter m is the mean of the observations. Prove that this is also the maximum likelihood estimator.

2. Consider a double intercross of the type $AB/ab \times AB/ab$ which produces the following numbers of offspring for the distinguishable phenotypes:

AB	Ab	aB	ab
187	35	37	31

    Find the maximum likelihood estimate of the recombination frequency (assume it's the same in the two sexes). What is the variance of your estimate?

3. You want to estimate the frequency of a particular transcript in a cDNA library. You plate out aliquots of the library (10^4 bacteria per plate), transfer the colonies to filters, hybridize to your probe, and count the number of spots on each filter. For a set of 10 filters you obtain the following results:

    $$15\ \ 23\ \ 20\ \ 20\ \ 17\ \ 13\ \ 22\ \ 22\ \ 27\ \ 19$$

    What is the mean transcript frequency (copies/10^4 clones) and what are its 95% confidence limits?

4. You are studying a series of promoter mutants by transfecting promoter/reporter constructs into cells and measuring reporter gene activity. You want to express the data as the ratio (R) between the mutant and control (wild type) values and have performed three independent experiments. Using the data below, compute the mean value for R and its standard deviation.

Mutant	Activity
control	87, 94, 68
m1	41, 42, 31
m2	153, 117, 182
m3	5, 21, 11

5. You have measured the diameters of a collection of perfectly spherical seeds and want to report the mean volume of the seeds. Based on the material above regarding the expectations and variances of functions, derive an approximate formula for the mean and variance of the volume in terms of the mean and variance of the measured diameters. For the following data set of diameters, use this approximate formula to estimate the mean and variance of the volume and compare these values to what you would get if you computed the volume for each seed and calculated the mean and variance using these calculated volumes. Values for the diameters are 125, 189, 334, 110, 48, and 99.

4. HYPOTHESIS AND SIGNIFICANCE TESTING

A scientific hypothesis makes a testable statement about the observable universe. A statistical hypothesis is more restricted in that it concerns the behavior of a measurable (or observable) random variable. Much of the work that we do is directed toward rephrasing a scientific hypothesis in terms that allow us to construct an appropriate statistical hypothesis. Say that we are concerned with a random variable x which falls in a sample space W. We can define (at our choosing) a subregion of the sample space, w. Since x is a random variable whose behavior in W is governed by a probability distribution, we can compute the probability that x will fall within our subregion w (*i.e.*, $P(x \in w)$). Any hypothesis concerning $P(x \in w)$ is a statistical hypothesis.

4.1. The Hypothesis Test

We will begin our discussion of statistical tests with a brief description of the classical *hypothesis test* scheme developed by Jerzy Neyman and E.S. Pearson in a series of classic papers published in the 1930's (reviewed by Lehman, 1993). Although this approach is perhaps more appropriate to industrial applications and quality control situations than to science, it is fairly easy to understand at the basic level and includes important concepts that carry over into the somewhat looser approach of *significance tests* that we will follow in this book.

A Neyman-Pearson hypothesis test may be described as comprising four elements:

1. A *null* hypothesis.

2. An *alternative* hypothesis.

3. A *partitioning* of the sample space (the set of all possible experimental outcomes) into two regions: the *acceptance* region and the *rejection* region.

4. A *decision* rule: If your experimental observation falls in the acceptance region, accept the null hypothesis as true, if the observation falls in the rejection region, reject the null hypothesis in favor of the alternative hypothesis.

These four elements are to be decided upon before you do your experiment and the conclusion of the whole process is meant to be a decision—thumbs up or thumbs down. Now, even in this rather rigid setup, we should not take too seriously the terms *accept* and *reject*— they are technical terms within the theory, but should not be interpreted too literally. In science we never completely accept without reservation an hypothesis as true.

Example 4.1

Suppose our experiment is to determine the sex ratio in a particular cross yielding 10 progeny; let π be the true probability of a female (F) and 1-π the true probability of a male (M). We know that either the cross has a normal sex ratio (π= 0.5), or it is biased in favor of females with $\pi = 0.8$. Admittedly, this is a bit artificial, but it will allow us to discuss all the more important concepts without getting tangled up in a morass of complex calculations.

1. Null hypothesis: $\pi = 0.5$
2. Alternate hypothesis: $\pi = 0.8$
3. Acceptance region: Number of F's observed in set $\{0,1,2,3,4,5,6,7\}$,
    Rejection region: Number of F's observed in set $\{8,9,10\}$.
4. Decision rule: We collect and sex our 10 progeny. If the number of F's is ≤ 7, we accept the cross as normal; if the number of F's is >7, we reject the idea of a normal sex ratio in favor of the hypothesis that the ratio is biased and $\pi=0.8$.

Is this a reasonable procedure? What properties should a reasonable procedure have?

First of all, it should be clear that in any finite experiment, we can never be 100% sure whether we have a "0.5" cross or a "0.8" cross. If there were a way of determining that type without error, the problem would not be a statistical one. That consideration leads to the first set of important concepts:

Type I error: The probability, α, of rejecting the null hypothesis when it is true.

Type II error: The probability, β, of accepting the null hypothesis when it is false

In our example,

$$\alpha = \sum_{h=8}^{10} \binom{10}{h} 0.5^{10} = 0.0547$$

$$\beta = \sum_{h=0}^{7} \binom{10}{h} 0.8^{h} \, 0.2^{10-h} = 0.3222$$

We find that we will commit a Type I error about 5% of the time, a reasonable rate of error; but that we will incorrectly accept the null hypothesis when, in fact, the cross is biased almost 1/3 of the time. That result doesn't seem very satisfactory and leads to the next important concept:

The *power* of a test: The *power* is the probability of rejecting the null hypothesis when it is false, *i.e.*, 1 - β.

In our case the power is about 2/3 – not very impressive. The reason, of course, is that the sample is quite small. In all hypothesis tests, there is always a trade-off between α and β. If you lower α, then β will increase, and *vice versa*. The only way to increase the power for a fixed α, is to increase the sample size (or find a better test).

4.2. The Significance Test

There is a slightly different way of approaching the same problem. Instead of thinking of it as a decision problem, we simply construct a measure of how well the data agree with the null hypothesis. Much of the reasoning is very similar to the Neyman-Pearson approach, but the outlook is somewhat different. Throughout the rest of this book we will tend to favor this approach.

We assign to each possible outcome of the experiment a *significance level* or *P-value*. This value is a number between 0 and 1 that indicates how well the data conform to the assumptions of the null hypothesis. This approach involves two operations:

1. Ordering all possible outcomes from least significant to most significant. (The ordering may be partial.)

2. Assigning P-values to each outcome such that more significant (less supportive of the null hypothesis) outcomes receive smaller P-values.

If we don't utilize any particular alternate hypothesis, the process leads to what is sometimes called a *pure* test of significance. Generally, however, there is some alternate hypothesis in mind, and it aids us in how we order the possible outcomes.

A reasonable (but not unique) procedure would be as follows:

1. Order the possible outcomes according to the likelihood ratio

$$\frac{L(outcome \,|\, H_1)}{L(outcome \,|\, H_0)}$$

Outcomes with higher ratios being deemed more significant than those with smaller ratios.

2. Evaluate the P-value of each outcome, x, as the sum of the probabilities, under the null hypothesis, of all outcomes at least as significant as x according to the above ordering.

3. Do the experiment, observe the outcome, and report the P-value for the observed outcome. For example, if $P=0.61$, the data evidently are in reasonable conformity with the null hypothesis. However, if $P=0.003$, then doubt is raised as to the validity of the null hypothesis and the alternate hypothesis starts looking more appealing. You may well still have some cutoff point, like $P=0.05$, in mind, at which point you start to doubt the null hypothesis and prefer the alternative, but that is not an intrinsic part of this approach.

Below is the calculation of the significance test P-values for Example 4.1. Notice the close similarity to the hypothesis testing scheme in this simple example. Our rejection region in that scheme was {8,9,10 females} and these three events, indeed correspond to the outcomes with the three smallest *P*-values. However, in our attempt to define a rejection region with probability around 5%, we left out of it the outcome F=7, which according to the likelihood ratio is actually more favorable to the alternative hypothesis! So the Neyman-Pearson approach would have obliged us to accept the null hypothesis based on an observed outcome (7 females) that really argues for the alternative hypothesis. Anomalies like this often come up especially when dealing with discrete distributions.

Example 4.1 (*cont.*)

F	$P(F \mid H_0)$	$P(F \mid H_1)$	Likelihood Ratio	P-value
0	0.0010	0.0000	0.0001	1.000
1	0.0098	0.0000	0.0004	0.9990
2	0.0439	0.0000	0.0017	0.9893
3	0.1172	0.0007	0.0067	0.9453
4	0.2051	0.0055	0.0268	0.8281
5	0.2461	0.0264	0.1074	0.6230
6	0.2050	0.0881	0.4295	0.3769
7	0.1172	0.2013	1.7179	0.1719
8	0.0439	0.3020	6.8719	0.0547
9	0.0098	0.2684	27.487	0.0107
10	0.0010	0.1074	109.9512	0.0010

Example 4.1 was picked for its simplicity in order to introduce basic concepts. Both of our hypotheses, null and alternative, were, in the jargon of statistics, *simple*; they each completely specified their corresponding probability distribution. Real testing problems, whichever approach is used, are generally more complex and involve so-called *composite* hypotheses.

4.3. Simple *versus* Composite Hypotheses

A probability distribution is often determined by the values of a set of parameters. A *simple* statistical hypothesis specifies a unique value for each parameter of the distribution. For example, we may wish to test the hypothesis that a set of observations comes from a Poisson distribution with a mean of 4.0. This hypothesis is simple because it specifies the sole parameter for the distribution and thus the entire distribution. Alternatively, we may wish to compare two sets of observations and test the hypothesis that the two sets come from the same Poisson distribution with mean m, m unspecified. Since we don't care what the value of m is but only that a single value can account for both of the sample distributions, this hypothesis is *composite*. In general, if a random variable follows a probability distribution with r parameters and our hypothesis specifies k of these parameters, the hypothesis is simple if $r = k$ and is composite if $r > k$. Most of the rest of the course will be devoted to defining statistical tests of various types, with composite alternative hypotheses.

Example 4.2

A first approach to discerning developmentally detrimental effects of genes that have an easily observed dominant phenotype is to determine whether the number of progeny homozygous for the gene in a cross between heterozygotes is smaller than would be predicted by Mendelian segregation. Suppose that we have isolated a mutant, D, and, to make matters simple, we can determine all three genotypes (D/D, $D/+$, and $+/+$) by virtue of an RFLP on Southern blots or PCR analysis. We mate two $D/+$ animals and determine the genotypes of 20 of the progeny. We find that 2 are D/D, 12 are $D/+$ and 6 are $+/+$.

4.4. Choosing the Null and Alternative Hypotheses

Prior to doing the above experiment, we should have a scientific hypothesis in mind, the nature of which will play a role in how we perform our experiment. We could construct a variety of scientific hypotheses, some of which are stated below.

S_1:   As stated in Example 4.2 the hypothesis of interest is that the mutant gene D has a detrimental effect during development in its homozygous state such that "few" D/D embryos survive to term.

S_2:   The allele D has developmentally detrimental effects, such that both D/D and $D/+$ offspring are underrepresented.

S_3: Segregation of the D and $+$ alleles is non-Mendelian.

The first step toward testing any of the above is to decide on the nature of the random variable to be measured and to determine its probability distribution under some defined (and relevant to our scientific hypothesis) set of conditions. For any of the above, we could look at the number of D/D progeny obtained, although this random variable might not be the best choice in all circumstances. Note that these three scientific hypotheses make quite different assertions about the numbers of each genotype that would occur. In spite of these distinctions, the contrary, or null hypothesis, is the same, *i.e.*, the number of D/D progeny is binomially distributed with a success probability of $p = 0.25$.

$$H_0: p = 0.25$$

In the cases of S_1 and S_2 above, we are interested in the same composite alternative hypothesis

$$H_{A1}: p < 0.25$$

that is, the D/D class is underrepresented. Note that this approach to asking S_2 does not take into account all of the useful information (the number of $D/+$ progeny is not specifically considered) and our hypothesis test is not optimal. In the case of S_3, we are interested in a more general composite alternative hypothesis

$$H_{A2}: p \neq 0.25$$

and again we are not making optimal use of the available information. Comparisons between H_0 and H_{A1} are said to be *one-sided* tests while that between H_0 and H_{A2} is a *two-sided* test.

4.5. Performing the Statistical Test

Now it would seem that we have to decide whether we are going to perform a hypothesis test or a significance test. To be honest, most scientists (and statisticians too!) do not always make a clear distinction between the two; probably because they usually involve largely the same calculations and tend to lead one to the same conclusion.

4.5.1. The hypothesis test approach.

To construct an hypothesis test, we first specify the null hypothesis, H_0, and then decide on a value of α, the Type I error rate. This value, also referred to as the significance level or *size* of the test, will typically be fairly small (*e.g.*, 0.05) so that we don't often make a Type I error. We then determine the set of outcomes (the critical or rejection region), with a combined probability of α, that will cause us to reject the null hypothesis. If our observed result falls within this set of outcomes, we reject the null hypothesis, otherwise we accept it.

4.5.2. The significance test approach.

Here we just calculate the *P*-value that corresponds to our observed outcome. How we view that value, *i.e.*, what we "do" after seeing it and thinking about it, is not really a formal part of the theory. Usually our behavior will be very similar to the Neyman-Pearson decision-maker, but we are not formally bound by our approach to make any particular decision.

4.5.3. A complication arising out of composite hypotheses.

Whichever approach we are inclined to use, a complication has arisen in Example 4.2 that was not present in Example 4.1. In Example 4.2, the alternative hypothesis is composite—the alternate hypothesis is a set (actually an interval) of values of the binomial probability, not one particular value. So now how do we use the alternative hypothesis to calculate Neyman-Pearson power or to order our outcomes for a significance test?

The power question is fairly straightforward. Clearly there is now no single power for our test of the hypothesis, but a different power for each possible value of the binomial probability included in the alternative hypothesis. The power is a function rather than a single value. This function is described in detail in the next section for Example 4.2.

If we are significance test animals, and are using the likelihood ratio method to order our outcomes, how do we do it when the alternative is composite? Obviously,

$$\frac{L(outcome \,|\, H_1)}{L(outcome \,|\, H_0)}$$

no longer specifies a unique number for each outcome because H_1 refers to a set of values of the binomial probability. The method most often used is to order the outcomes according to

$$\frac{\max_{p \in H_1} L(outcome | H_1)}{L(outcome | H_0)}$$

the maximum being taken over all values of the binomial probability in H_1.

In any event, it is useful to provide a rough verbal definition of the meaning of the *P-value* obtained in such a test:

> *The significance level, or P-value, is the probability of obtaining the observed result or a more extreme result (one less consistent with the null hypothesis) under the assumption that the null hypothesis is true.*

Left unspecified in this definition, of course, is exactly what is meant by "more extreme," and whether or not its definition makes use of an alternative hypothesis or not. In our example we used a likelihood ratio criterion; but others are possible. The most obvious is simply the difference $|p - p_0|$ where p_0 is the value of the binomial probability assigned by the null hypothesis and p denotes the value(s) assigned by the alternate hypothesis. Another possibility is simply to order the possible outcomes by their probabilities under the null hypothesis as is done in the so-called "pure" test of significance (this method, of course, doesn't take into account any specific alternative hypothesis).

In Example 4.2, the test of the null hypothesis

$$H_0: \; p = 0.25$$

against the alternative

$$H_{A1}: \; p < 0.25$$

would be obtained by summing the probabilities of obtaining 0, 1, and 2 *D/D* progeny for a binomial distribution with $N = 20$ and $p = 0.25$. These probabilities are 0.00317, 0.0211, and 0.0669, respectively, giving us a significance level of $P = 0.091$. This *P*-value may be interpreted as a sort of inverse measure of the confidence with which we can discard the null hypothesis in favor of our alternative. Although it is customary to use a *P*-value of 0.05 (or less) to reject the null hypothesis (the hypothesis test approach), the choice of this value is arbitrary. In our case, we could interpret the results of this experiment to say that we are suspicious (if not entirely convinced) that D/D animals are lost during development (the significance test approach), and it would be reasonable at this point to do another experiment to cause us to tilt one way or the other on the question.

4.5.4. Choosing between one-sided and two-sided tests.

In the example above, we discussed testing the same null hypothesis (i.e., $p = 0.25$) against either a one-sided ($p < 0.25$) or a two-sided ($p \neq 0.25$) alternative, depending on the biological question we were asking. It will likely have occurred to you that a one-sided test will give a smaller P-value (generally half) when the deviation is in the "desired" direction than the two-sided test. As discussed below (Chapter 10), it will also have greater power, since you're only looking at half of the sample space. You should avoid the temptation of routinely performing one-sided tests (in the direction of your preconceived idea of how the experiment should work out). When you do so, you are asserting that you would have *absolutely no interest* in pursuing further studies if your results pointed in the other direction. Thus, for most of the experiments you do, performing a two-sided test would be more appropriate. However, there are some questions that are intrinsically one-sided. For example, you want to test whether a specific chemical causes cancer and might pose a health risk to people. You treat groups of mice with the chemical or a vehicle control and after an appropriate period of time, you assess the incidence of cancer at a particular organ site. Because of the reason you are doing the experiment (safety testing), a one-sided test of whether the incidence in treated mice exceeds that in control mice would be entirely appropriate.

4.6. The Power of Statistical Tests

The concept of power comes out of the hypothesis testing scheme. The idea, as we saw above, is to set the size of the test and then look for a test with the greatest power.

One way of looking at the above example is that we simply didn't do a large enough experiment to detect an effect of the D/D genotype on viability. Before doing an experiment, it is useful to consider the power, the chance that our experiment will detect an effect, of the statistical test we plan to use. In this case, the power is simply $1 - \beta$, the complement of the probability of making a Type II error. Unlike the Type I error probability, which we can view as being fixed by the investigator, the probability for a Type II error depends on both the value of α that we consider acceptable (that is, the largest value of α that would cause us to reject the null hypothesis) and on the degree of deviation from the null hypothesis that we would like to be able to detect (in this case, the largest value of the frequency of D/D offspring that we would find interesting). We will spend more time on this problem later (Chapter 10), but for our simple example we can compute the power of the experiment fairly easily.

Example 4.2 continued

In our example, say that we would like to fix α at 0.05 and be able to detect a reduction in the frequency of D/D progeny under the alternative hypothesis to 0.1 (as against the null hypothesis value of 0.25). We can compute the power $(1 - \beta)$ of the experiment as a function of N as follows. For a given value of N, we can determine the *critical value* of x, the number of D/D offspring, that would allow us to reject the null hypothesis with a significance level of at most 0.05. For $N = 20$, using the binomial probabilities given above we would reject the null hypothesis only in the cases that the number of D/D offspring was less than or equal to 1, since $P(x \leq 1) = 0.024$ and $P(x \leq 2) = 0.091$. Thus, the critical value of x is 1 for $N = 20$. Under the alternative hypothesis that the proportion of D/D progeny is 0.1, we can use a binomial distribution with $N = 20$, $p = 0.1$ to calculate the probability of 1 or fewer D/D animals as 0.391. Thus, the power of our experiment to detect a frequency of D/D animals less than or equal to 0.1 when $N = 20$ is 0.391. The table and figure below summarize power calculations for various values in this experiment. You can see from the table that in order to have a greater than 90% probability of detecting the desired alternative we would require a sample size of about 55 progeny.

N	Critical value (α=0.05)	Power
15	0	0.206
20	1	0.391
30	3	0.647
40	5	0.794
50	7	0.877
60	9	0.926
70	11	0.956
80	13	0.973

4.7. Sample Problems

1. It seems reasonable to suppose that the more lethal the D/D genotype, the fewer progeny must be analyzed to demonstrate a deviation from Mendelian segregation. If we use a binomial probability of $p=0.01$ for our alternative hypothesis, what is the power of an experiment involving the analysis of 20 offspring? Assume that all of the other parameters of the above example are the same: the binomial probability under the null hypothesis is $p=0.25$, and the desired value for the significance level is $\alpha=0.05$.

2. Again using the above example, consider the case in which the survival of both the D/D and D/d progeny is reduced relative to the d/d offspring. You do an experiment mating D/d parents and examine the genotypes of 20 offspring. You observe that 2 are D/D, 9 are D/d, and 9 are d/d in genotype. There are two alternative tests using the binomial distribution to compare these results to the expected proportions of 0.25:0.5:0.25, depending on whether you test for the presence of too few D/D offspring or too many d/d offspring. What significance level (P-value) do you obtain for each test? In the case that the survival of D/D offspring is 10% and that for D/d offspring is 50% (with that for d/d being 100%), what is the power of each test when 20 offspring are analyzed and an $\alpha = 0.05$ is used?

5. TESTING FOR DIFFERENCES IN LOCATION

The most commonly encountered statistical problem is that of testing for differences in location between measurements made on two independent populations. We are accustomed to thinking of this problem as testing for a difference in the mean values for the two populations but we could also phrase the problem in a slightly different way. For example, we might ask whether a randomly chosen member of population 1 is likely to be larger in magnitude than a randomly chosen member of population 2. The classical normal theory test for a difference in the mean (μ) of two normally distributed random variables is the Student t-test, which defines a test statistic

$$t_v = \frac{\overline{x}_1 - \overline{x}_2}{\left\{\left[\frac{(n_1-1)s_1^2 + (n_2-1)s_2^2}{n_1+n_2-2}\right]\left(\frac{n_1+n_2}{n_1 n_2}\right)\right\}^{1/2}}$$

where $\overline{x}_i$ is the mean for group i, s_i^2 is the variance, n_i is the number of observations, and v, the number of degrees of freedom, is n_1+n_2-2.

The null hypothesis, that $\overline{x}_1$ is equal to $\overline{x}_2$, is rejected for large or small (negative) values of the statistic. Although this familiar statistic is easy to compute, the two assumptions required for using this test are often violated by data from biological experiments. First, the test is quite sensitive to "heavy tails" in the distribution for the data. The frequency of observations for normally distributed data falls off rapidly as the value becomes much less than or greater than the mean value, making the test sensitive to outlier or extreme values. Second, the assumption that the variances for the two populations are equal and essentially independent of the mean values for the populations is contrary to the dependence of the variance on the mean for many simple distributions (*e.g.*, Poisson) of biological interest.

5.1. Permutation Tests

The second version of the location question posed above, that randomly chosen members of population 1 are likely to be larger than those from population 2, provides the rationale for an alternative approach based on examining all possible permutations of the observed data set.

Consider the following small experiment, in which we make three independent observations under each of two conditions:

Group A: 29, 52, 49

Group B: 15, 36, 18

We want to test the null hypothesis that there is no difference in "location" between the two treatments against the one-sided alternative that the observations in group A are larger than those in group B. We observed that the mean of group A (m_A) is 43.3 and that for group B is 23; thus, we could define a statistic for testing our hypothesis, $D = m_A - m_B$, which is equal to 20.3 for the above case.

A (m_A)	B (m_B)	D	A (m_A)	B (m_B)	D
29,52,49 (43.3)	15,36,18 (23)	20.3	52,49,15 (38.7)	29,36,18 (27.7)	11
29,52,15 (32)	49,36,18 (34.3)	-2.3	52,49,36 (45.7)	29,15,18 (20.7)	25
29,52,36 (39)	49,15,18 (27.3)	11.7	52,49,18 (39.7)	29,15,36 (26.7)	13
29,52,18 (33)	49,15,36 (33.3)	-0.3	52,15,36 (34.3)	29,49,18 (32)	2.3
29,49,15 (31)	52,36,18 (35.3)	-4.3	52,15,18 (28.3)	29,49,36 (38)	-9.7
29,49,36 (38)	52,15,18 (28.3)	9.7	52,36,18 (35.3)	29,49,15 (31)	4.3
29,49,18 (32)	52,15,36 (34.3)	-2.3	49,15,36 (33.3)	29,52,18 (33)	0.3
29,15,36 (26.7)	52,49,18 (39.7)	-13	49,15,18 (27.3)	29,52,36 (39)	-11.7
29,15,18 (20.7)	52,49,36 (45.7)	-25	49,36,18 (34.3)	29,52,15 (32)	2.3
29,36,18 (27.7)	52,49,15 (38.7)	-11	15,36,18 (23)	29,52,49 (43.3)	-20.3

Under the null hypothesis that the two sets of observations come from the same population, we could randomly draw any three of the six observations and label them as "A". The distribution of our test statistic, D, can be computed for all $\binom{6}{3} = 20$ permutations of the data set. The significance level for our hypothesis test can then be obtained by dividing the number of permutations for which $D \geq 20.3$ by the total number of permutations, 20. The 20 permutations of our data set, and the corresponding value of our test statistic, are enumerated in the table above. From the table, you can see that only 2 permutations give test statistics that equal or exceed our observed value, 20.3. Thus, the P-value for our one-sided statistical test is 0.1. If we had been testing against a two-sided alternative hypothesis, we would count the number of permutations for which $|D| \geq 20.3$ (4 in this case).

The above permutation test has the advantage that it provides an exact test of our hypothesis without requiring us to make any assumptions about the underlying model that generated the data (*e.g.*, the assumption of normality in the *t*-test). This approach can be applied quite generally as long as we can define an appropriate test statistic. For example, we might be interested in comparing two analytical methods for their precision in measuring some parameter and we've made multiple observations using each method for the same sample. To test for a difference in precision, we could define a test statistic $D = V(A) - V(B)$, where $V(x)$ is the variance of x.

5.1.1. Monte Carlo methods.

A major disadvantage to the permutation test above is that the magnitude of the computational problem scales up very rapidly with the sample size. The numbers of permutations that we would have to enumerate for two groups of 3, 5, 10, and 20 observations each are 20, 252, 184756, and 1.37847×10^{11}.

The complete set of permutations defines the sample space for our statistical test under the null hypothesis. One way of thinking about our hypothesis test is that we want to know what fraction of the points in the sample space would provide a test statistic that equals or exceeds our observed result. In the case that the sample space is very large, it is possible to estimate this fraction (our *P*-value) by simply examining a suitably large number of randomly chosen points within the sample space. This approach falls under the general heading of "Monte Carlo" methods. Given access to a desktop computer and with a little programming, this approach can be used as generally as the strict permutation test described above.

Example 5.1

We are studying the induction of cell proliferation in a target tissue following treatment of animals with a particular chemical. We treat groups of 14 and 13 animals with the agent or solvent vehicle, respectively, along with BUdR to label replicating cells. Animals are sacrificed, the tissue is prepared, and we examine 10,000 cells from each animal and count the number of labeled cells. We obtained the following data:

Treated: 563, 504, 837, 262, 435, 283, 218, 1296, 1310, 1311, 658, 426, 794, 297
Control: 231, 79, 290, 119, 346, 493, 349, 299, 747, 121, 109, 204, 114.

The means and standard deviations for the treated and control groups are 657±399 and 269±189, respectively.

We want to test the null hypothesis that the levels of proliferation in treated and control animals are the same against the one-sided alternative that the treated animals show a higher labeling index. We can define a test statistic, $D = M_{treated} - M_{control}$, as the mean of the treated group minus the mean of the control group.

Our sample space under the null hypothesis consists of more than 20 million points. We decide to use a Monte Carlo approach and run 100,000 random trials on our data set and compute the value of D for each (at the cost of about a half hour of programming and one minute of computation). The complement (upper tail) of the cumulative distribution for the test statistic is shown in the figure below. Our observed test statistic is 388 and the fraction of trials for which $D \geq 388$ is approximately 0.001, which is our P-value for the statistical test.

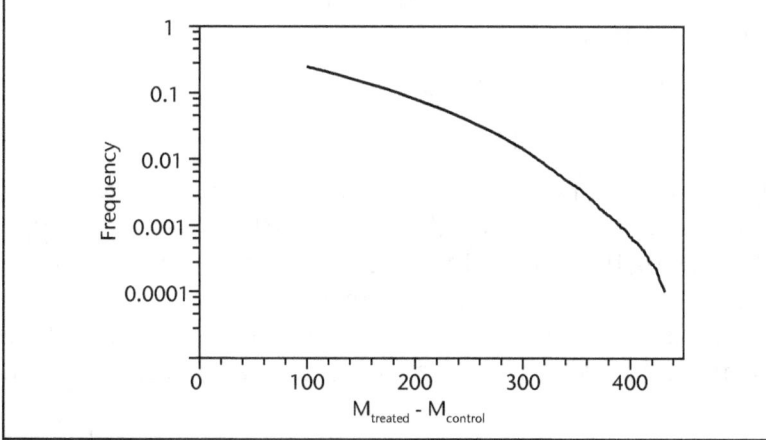

5.2. Wilcoxon Rank Sum Test

The permutation tests described above require that we define (or approximate) a unique distribution for our test statistic for every experiment. A much more convenient approach is to base the statistical tests on the ranks (or ordered magnitudes) of the observations rather than on the observed values. As will become evident, this approach requires very few assumptions concerning the distribution(s) followed by the data and hence the methods are often referred to as distribution-free or nonparametric tests. A further advantage to tests based on ranks is that they are relatively insensitive to the presence of extreme values (outliers) in the samples.

5.2.1. Rationale and a simple example.

Consider an experiment to test the ability of a particular gene to confer the property of anchorage-independent growth on a mammalian cell line that normally has a low frequency of colony formation when cultured in semisolid medium. Two plasmid constructions, "A", which contains an antibiotic resistance marker, and "B", which is identical to the

"A" plasmid except that it also includes the test gene, are each introduced into populations of cells. Those cells that express antibiotic resistance (and hence carry the A or B DNA) are selected and samples of 10^4 cells are plated in semisolid medium. In this small experiment, 4 independent plates of "A" cells and 2 of "B" cells are scored for the number of colonies after a suitable period of time. The following data (number of colonies / 10^4 cells) are obtained:

A plasmid: 32 24 28 40

B plasmid: 116 120

The null hypothesis of interest is that the observations for the two groups of data come from identical populations against an alternative hypothesis that cells carrying the B plasmid are more likely to grow in agarose. If the null hypothesis were true, we might imagine that the second sample (B plasmid) could consist of any 2 of the 6 observations made in the experiment and that all possible permutations of the data would be equally likely.

Because we are only interested in the range of possible permutations of the data observed in the two groups, the actual values are irrelevant and we can consider just the ranks of the observations (from 1 to 6, smallest to largest). Replacing the observed values by their ranks (with the data in the same order as above)

A plasmid: 3 1 2 4

B plasmid: 5 6

It is convenient to have a single value or statistic derived from the data that gives a consistent measure of the relative magnitude of the observations in the sample. The simplest such statistic would be the sum of the ranks for the sample; for example, 11 in the case of the B plasmid.

The $\binom{6}{2} = 15$ possible permutations of the data for the B plasmid

sample along with the statistic are given in the table below. We can then tabulate the distribution under the null hypothesis for the rank sum statistic for the case of two samples of 4 and 2 observations. Each of the 15 permutations is equally likely (with frequency 1/15) under the null hypothesis.

In the case of our small experiment, the statistic for the observed data is equal to 11. From the distribution of the statistic under the null hypothesis, the probability of obtaining a rank sum this large (it can not in fact be larger) is 0.067.

This approach to the two-sample location problem is generally referred to as the Wilcoxon rank sum test (Wilcoxon, 1945). Permutation tests for differences in location, such as the Wilcoxon rank sum test, have the advantage of requiring few assumptions concerning the distribution of the data obtained in an experiment. The broad applicability of these tests exacts a relatively small cost in power (that is, they generally require only a few more observations) when compared with parametric tests that are based on explicit knowledge of the form of the distribution of the data. In this chapter, we will provide a more formal description of the Wilcoxon rank sum test and discuss analogous approaches to testing for differences in location in blocked data and for multiple samples.

5.2.2. Wilcoxon rank sum test—formal description.

Data and assumptions: Observations are taken on two independent groups. The first group consists of n observations X_i ($i=1 \ldots n$) and the second consists of m observations Y_j

Permutations		
B sample ranks		**Rank sum**
6	5	11
6	4	10
6	3	9
6	2	8
6	1	7
5	4	9
5	3	8
5	2	7
5	1	6
4	3	7
4	2	6
4	1	5
3	2	5
3	1	4
2	1	3

Rank Sum Distribution	
Sum	**Frequency**
11	1/15 (0.067)
10	1/15 (0.067)
9	2/15 (0.133)
8	2/15 (0.133)
7	3/15 (0.2)
6	2/15 (0.133)
5	2/15 (0.133)
4	1/15 (0.067)
3	1/15 (0.067)

(j=1 ... m). Without loss of generality, we can assume that $n \leq m$. Within each group the observations are assumed to be mutually independent and the X_i are assumed to come from a population with continuous cumulative distribution $F(x)$ while the Y_j are from a distribution $F(y)$. We want to test the null hypothesis

$$H_0: \ F(x) = F(y)$$

against either the two-sided alternative

$$H_2: \ F(x) \neq F(y)$$

or one-sided alternatives

$$H_1: \ F(x) < F(y) \text{ or } F(x) > F(y)$$

Test statistic: The n+m observations are assigned ranks from 1 to (n+m). The test statistic W_X is

$$W_X = \sum_{i=1}^{n} R_i$$

where R_i is the rank of the observation i.

The exact significance level for the appropriate alternative hypotheses can be obtained from the table in Appendix 4 as follows.

For the one sided hypothesis $F(x) < F(y)$ (*i.e.*, the X's are larger) enter the appropriate place in the table with x=W_X.

For the one-sided hypothesis $F(x) > F(y)$ (*i.e.*, the Y's are larger) enter the appropriate place in the table with the value x=[$n(m+n+1)-W_X$].

The distribution of the test statistic under the null hypothesis is symmetrical, so the significance level for the two-sided test is most simply obtained by doubling the P-value for the appropriate one-sided alternative.

Alternative form of the statistic: Recall that one of the ways to phrase the location question is in terms of the probability that a randomly chosen X-value will be larger than a randomly chosen Y-value. An equivalent statistic to the one described above, the Mann-Whitney (Mann and Whitney, 1947) statistic can be defined as

$$U_{XY} = \text{number of pairs for which } (X_i > Y_j)$$

such that U_{XY}/nm is the probability stated above. This is equivalent to the statistic given above since

$$W_X = U_{XY} + [n(n+1)/2]$$

Large-sample approximation: In cases where the number of observations exceeds the table for the Wilcoxon rank sum statistic, we can take advantage of the fact that, for large numbers of n and m observations, the statistic W_X is approximately normally distributed. The expected value for the statistic is

$$E(W_X) = n(n+m+1)/2$$

while the variance is

$$V(W_X) = nm(m+n+1)/12$$

We can thus define an approximate statistic

$$W^* = [W_X - E(W_X)] / V(W_X)^{1/2}$$

where W^* follows the standard normal distribution with mean of 0 and variance of 1. In the simple example given above, W_X was 11, n was 2 and m was 4. Thus, the approximate statistic would be

$$W^* = (11 - 7) / 4.67^{0.5} = 1.85$$

From the table of the standard normal distribution, this would correspond to a *P*-value of 0.032 which rather overstates the true significance level of 0.067. Applying a continuity correction in this case (*i.e.*, subtracting 0.5 from the numerator) improves the approximation and gives a *P*-value of 0.053. For values of n and m where both exceed 6 or so, the normal approximation is quite good, with or without a continuity correction.

Correction for tied observations: One of the assumptions made above was that the X_i and Y_j came from continuous distributions. Thus, there is no chance that any two values will be identical (*i.e.*, tied). However, all measurement data are at some level discrete and some experiments necessarily give rise to discretely distributed data. In the case where two or more observations in the experiment have identical values, the "exact" significance level obtained from the table for the W_X statistic is conservative. We could, of course, obtain an exact significance level by recomputing the null distribution for the test statistic as we did in our simple example, but in that case the result would be conditional for the observed pattern of tied values in the observations. The normal approximation described above remains unconditional in the presence of ties as long as we correct for the presence of tied groups of values.

Consider the following data set

>   Group 1: 5 8 10 12

>   Group 2: 4 0 5

We can rank the observations as before, except that average ranks (mid-ranks) will be assigned to tied values. The ranks are thus

>   Group 1: 3.5 5 6 7

>   Group 2: 2 1 3.5

The test statistic (Group 2) in this case is $W_X = 6.5$. The expected value for the test statistic, $E(W_X)$, remains unchanged when some of the values are tied, but the value of the variance decreases (since the number of possible values of the statistic is reduced) by an amount depending on the number of tied values.

$$V(W_X) = \left(\frac{nm}{(n+m)(n+m-1)} \sum_{i=1}^{n+m} R_i^2 \right) - \frac{nm(n+m+1)^2}{4(n+m-1)}$$

Note that this is identical to the variance given above when there are no ties. According to Lehman (1998), the continuity correction should not be applied to the normal approximation when the data set contains tied values.

Examples 5.2

A. Consider an experiment identical to the one for our transformation example above, but with a larger number of observations. The data are

>   A plasmid: 70 55 80 140
>   B plasmid: 116 220 405 410 550 735

We wish to test the null hypothesis that the two plasmids yield the same colony forming efficiency against the one-sided alternative that the plating efficiency of the cells carrying the A plasmid is smaller. The ranks for the observations are

> A plasmid: 2 1 3 5
> B plasmid: 4 6 7 8 9 10

Thus, the value of the test statistic is W_x=11. We can enter the table using the value x=44-11=33, which indicates a P-value of 0.0095. Note that in this case, the normal approximation would give W*= -2.34 for an approximate P-value of 0.0095.

B. In Example 5.1, we used Monte Carlo methods to compare the BUdR labeling index for tissue from control animals and those treated with a test chemical. Ranking the observations for the two groups we obtain

Treated: 20, 19, 24, 9, 17, 10, 7, 25, 26, 27, 21, 16, 23, 12
Control: 8, 1, 11, 4, 14, 18, 15, 13, 22, 5, 2, 6, 3

The sum of the ranks for the treated group is 256. Using the normal approximation, we obtain

$$W^* = (256 - 196)/(424.67)^{0.5} = 2.912$$

From Appendix 1, the one-sided P-value is 0.0018, similar to the significance level we obtained by our Monte Carlo approach.

We can use midranks and the approximate statistic in a useful way for constructing a one-sided test in a $2 \times t$ contingency table (see Chapter 6) where the t columns differ in an ordered way.

Example 5.3

We are interested in a gene *a* that we believe causes a variety of developmental defects when present in the homozygous state in the animal. The effect of the gene is pleiotropic but generally doesn't interfere with our ability to produce *Aa* and *aa* progeny. A number of individuals of each genotype are evaluated by an outside observer (who doesn't know the genotype) and classified according to whether the animals are normal, or defective to a mild, moderate, or severe extent. We obtain the following data

Genotype		Defect			
	None	Mild	Moderate	Severe	Sum
Aa	2	10	4	2	18
aa	0	3	7	10	20
Sum	2	13	11	12	38

We could think of these data in terms of assigning a value of 0, 1, 2, or 3 to each animal according to the severity of its defect. The midranks for the individuals in each category would be

	None	Mild	Moderate	Severe
Midrank	1.5	9	21	32.5

We can compute the test statistic

$$W_X = 2(1.5) + 10(9) + 4(21) + 2(32.5) = 242$$

Using the normal approximation (and correcting for the ties), $W^* = -3.35$, or $P < 0.0004$.

5.3. Analysis of Paired Data

In some experiments we would like to analyze a treatment effect under conditions where we expect that uninteresting sources of variation may also operate. We can test for such a treatment effect in spite of confounding variation by blocking the data according to the suspected confounding variables. A simple case of this approach is provided by Problem 7 in section 2.5.

Each of the n samples in this type of experiment consists of two observations (X_i, Y_i) $(i=1...n)$ and we are interested in testing the null hypothesis

$$H_0: Z_i = Y_i - X_i = 0$$

against an appropriate one-sided or two-sided alternative. The Wilcoxon signed-rank test (Wilcoxon, 1945) provides a means of considering this hypothesis. For the one-sided alternative that the Y_i are larger than the X_i, we would expect that the magnitudes of the positive deviations (Z_i) would generally be larger than the negative deviations. Under the null hypothesis, each Z_i is equally likely to be positive or negative; thus, there are 2^n possible permutations of the ranks of the magnitudes of the Z_i. As before, we can define a test statistic based on the sum of a subset of the ranks *(e.g.,* the positive Z_i) and determine the null distribution of this test statistic by adding up the appropriate permutations.

5.3.1. Signed rank statistic.

To compute the statistic, determine the values of the n differences Z_i, and rank the absolute values of these differences from 1 to n to give R_i. If, for example, the number of negative ranks is smaller, compute the statistic as the sum of the ranks for which $Z_i < 0$.

$$W_s = \Sigma R_i \text{ for all } Z_i < 0.$$

The significance level can then be determined by consulting the table in Appendix 5 or by using the normal approximation given below. Samples for which $Z_i = 0$ are dropped from the analysis, reducing the value of n. In the case of tied values, midranks are used and the approximate procedure below should be used for determination of the significance level.

Large sample approximation and correction for ties: An alternative method for computing the signed rank statistic, suggested by Conover (1999), is convenient when the sample size is large or when ties are present in the Z_i. As above, samples for which $Z_i = 0$ are discarded, leaving n nonzero observations. The n samples are ranked according to the magnitude of the difference, $|Z_i|$, and for each sample, the value R_i is assigned as the above rank, but given the sign of the corresponding Z_i. The test statistic

$$T = \frac{\sum_{i=1}^{n} R_i}{\sqrt{\sum_{i=1}^{n} R_i^2}}$$

follows a standard normal distribution.

Example 5.4

Consider an experiment in which the level of transcription for a test plasmid is compared for a series of cell lines that have been constructed to express (or not express) a putative transactivating protein. Because we are generally interested in the ratio of expression, we will define the Z_i as $\log(Y_i)-\log(X_i)$. We obtain the following data

Line	RNA (Arbitrary units)		Z_i	Rank	R_i
	-transact.	+transact.			
1	20	30	+0.176	3	+3
2	14	35	+0.397	5	+5
3	47	46	-0.009	1	-1
4	5	50	+1.0	7	+7
5	11	9	-0.087	2	-2
6	6	18	+0.477	6	+6
7	8	16	+.301	4	+4

Because there are fewer negative values, we determine the sum of the ranks for $Z_i<0$ as

$$W_s = 1 + 2 = 3.$$

Entering the table in the appendix with the value 3, we obtain a P-value of 0.039.

Using the large sample approximation, we would obtain
$T = 1.859$ and a one-sided P-value of approximately 0.031.

5.4. Multiple Samples

The discussion above focused on simple experimental designs in which we were interested in testing for differences in location between two independent samples. Often our experiments will consist of three or more samples representing, *e.g.*, expression data for a series of mutant constructs or responses of animals to several different dose levels of a drug. We will discuss the problem of making inferences regarding various pair-wise combinations of treatment groups in Chapter 9. Tests based on sample ranks for the hypothesis that all of the groups in an experiment show the same response are described below.

5.4.1. A multisample test against a general alternative.

Our data consist of k samples, each with n_i observations with values x_{ij} ($i = 1 \dots k, j = 1 \dots n_i$). The total number of observations in our experiment is N, the sum of the n_i. We want to test the null hypothesis that all of the samples are taken from the same population against the alternative that at least one sample is drawn from a population with a different location from the others. The Kruskal-Wallis test is based on jointly ranking all N observations and determining whether the ranks are randomly distributed across the k samples (Kruskal and Wallis, 1952).

For each sample, i, compute the sum of the ranks

$$R_i = \sum_{j=1}^{n_i} r_{ij}$$

where r_{ij} is the rank of observation x_{ij} ($1 \le r_{ij} \le N$). When no ties are present among the x_{ij}, the Kruskal-Wallis test statistic, H, is

$$H = \left(\frac{12}{N(N+1)} \sum_{i=1}^{k} \frac{R_i^2}{n_i} \right) - 3(N+1)$$

which follows a χ^2 distribution with k-1 degrees of freedom. If some of the x_{ij} are tied, mid-ranks are used for the r_{ij} and R_i is computed as above. The test statistic, H, is

$$H = \frac{1}{S^2}\left[\left(\sum_{i=1}^{k}\frac{R_i^2}{n_i}\right) - \frac{N(N+1)^2}{4}\right] \quad \text{where}$$

$$S^2 = \frac{1}{N-1}\left[\left(\sum_{i=1}^{k}\sum_{j=1}^{n_i}r_{ij}^2\right) - \frac{N(N+1)^2}{4}\right]$$

Unless the number of ties is large, there will be little difference in the results for the two formulas for H.

Example 5.5

We have been studying the genetics of blood pressure in rats and have become concerned that the various diets used by our group and other labs working on hypertensive rats may affect the measured blood pressure. To test this hypothesis, we place groups of rats on three different diets and, after several weeks, measure the blood pressure for animals from each group. Our results are (mm Hg)

Diet 1
139 167 132 144 129 113 126 153 174 127 149 133

Diet 2
126 93 147 154 98 128 126 132 169 133

Diet 3
116 152 143 125 141 154 152 147 159 141 115 113
171 114 140 139 149 96 140 152

The ranks for these observations (using mid-ranks for tied values) are

Diet 1
20.5 39 16.5 27 15 4.5 11 35 42 13 30.5 18.5

Diet 2
11 1 28.5 36.5 3 14 11 16.5 40 18.5

Diet 3
8 33 26 9 24.5 36.5 33 28.5 38 24.5 7 4.5 41 6 22.5 20.5
30.5 2 22.5 33

The sums of the ranks for the three diets are 272.5, 180, and
450.5, respectively. The Kruskal-Wallis test statistic is approximately

$$H = \left(\frac{12}{42(42+1)} \times \left[\frac{272.5^2}{12} + \frac{180^2}{10} + \frac{450.5^2}{20} \right] \right) - 3(42+1)$$

$$= 1.070$$

Using the χ^2 distribution with 2 degrees of freedom, we obtain a *P*-value of 0.58 and conclude that the blood pressure
values do not differ for these three diets.

5.4.2. A multisample test against an ordered alternative.

In many experiments there is a natural ordering among the treatment groups, *e.g.*, in the case of a dose-response. In this case, we obtain
data for *s* groups, each consisting of n_i (*i*=1 ... *s*) observations and wish to
test the null hypothesis

$$H_0: \ F(X_1) = F(X_2) = F(X_3) = ... = F(X_s)$$

against the one-sided alternative (for example)

$$H_1: \ F(X_1) \geq F(X_2) \geq F(X_3) \geq ... \geq F(X_s)$$

(where at least one of the inequalities holds).

The Jonckheere-Terpstra test can be performed for this set of hypotheses as follows (Jonckheere, 1954):

Define the value

U_{ij} = number of $(X_{ia} < X_{jb})$ where $a=1...n_i$ and $b=1...n_j$

(Recall that this is the Mann-Whitney form of the rank sum statistic for the pair of samples i and j)

The Jonckheere-Terpstra statistic is computed using the $0.5(s)(s-1)$ values U_{ij} for $i<j$ as

$$U = \sum_{i<j} U_{ij}$$

Since the distribution of U depends on the pattern of the n_i, it is most convenient to use the usual normal approximation

$$U^* = [U-E(U)] / V(U)^{1/2}$$

where

$$E(U) = 0.25 \ (N^2 - \Sigma n_i^2)$$

$$V(U) = [N^2(2N+3) - \Sigma n_i^2(2n_i+3)] / 72$$

N is the total number of observations and the summation is over $i=1 ... s$.

In the case of tied observations, add $0.5 \times$ the number of ties in each i,j comparison to the value of U_{ij}. If there are g groups of tied values each of size t_k, the modified formula for the variance of U is

$$V(U) = \left\{ \frac{1}{72} \left[N(N-1)(2N+5) - \sum_{i=1}^{s} n_i(n_i-1)(2n_i+5) - \sum_{k=1}^{g} t_k(t_k-1)(2t_k+5) \right] \right.$$

$$+ \frac{1}{36N(N-1)(N-2)} \left[\sum_{i=1}^{s} n_i(n_i-1)(n_i-2) \right] \left[\sum_{k=1}^{g} t_k(t_k-1)(t_k-2) \right]$$

$$+ \left. \frac{1}{8N(N-1)} \left[\sum_{i=1}^{s} n_i(n_i-1) \right] \left[\sum_{k=1}^{g} t_k(t_k-1) \right] \right\}$$

As a final note, this test is most powerful when the treatment groups are, in some sense, equally spaced.

Example 5.6

We are studying a mutant gene that we suspect has a quantitative effect on male fertility. We collect a number of males (3 or 4) having 2, 1, or 0 copies of the mutant allele and mate each to 3 females. The observation for each male is the total number of progeny obtained in the matings.

i	Number of mutant alleles	Total number of progeny
1	2	16,8,6
2	1	27,16,15
3	0	31,29,18,42

We compute the values U_{ij} as

$$U_{12} = 7.5$$
$$U_{13} = 12$$
$$U_{23} = 11$$

For this example $U = 7.5 + 12 + 11 = 30.5$, $E(U) = 16.5$, and $V(U) = 27.25$. Thus, $U^* = 2.69$, giving a significance level of $P<0.0036$.

5.5. Sample Problems

1. There has been concern for some time that nitrite present in cured meats may result in the formation of carcinogenic N-nitrosamines in the stomach by reaction with amines in the diet. It is possible to safely measure the amount of nitrosamine production in humans by administering a large dose of proline and measuring the level of N-nitroso-proline, a non-toxic reaction product, excreted in the urine. You decide to test the hypothesis that eating a reasonable amount of a cured meat will increase the amount of nitrosation taking place in the stomach in the following way. Each of 6 subjects, who have been asked to avoid cured meats for the previous week, is given a dose of proline and the excretion of N-nitroso-proline is measured for 24 hours. Each subject is then fed a breakfast including 6 strips of bacon and a dose of proline; excretion of the nitrosated amino acid is again measured for 24 hours. You obtain the data listed below in the form (basal μg excreted, μg excreted after bacon).

   (3.1,2.8)   (2.0,6.1)   (5.1,4.5)   (4.2,2.9)
   (8.5,8.9)   (1.1,6.0)

   Did bacon consumption significantly increase the excretion of the N-nitroso-proline?

2. The recessive mutation *bg* (beige) in mice results in a decrease in the activity of natural killer cells in homozygous mutant mice. You test the hypothesis that this cell type plays an important role in rejection of tumor cells (derived from a tumor induced in an isogenic animal) by injecting animals with genotypes *bg/bg* or *bg/+* with 10^6 cells and measuring the time required for the development of a palpable tumor in each animal. You obtain the following data:

Genotype	Time to tumor development (days)
bg/+	28, 51, 47, 80
bg/bg	14, 35, 17, 37, 16

   Is there a significant difference in tumor latency between the two groups?

3. You have obtained data for four samples as follows:

Sample 1   32 24 28 40 0 15 20 55
Sample 2   20 36 5 15 30 25
Sample 3   35 25 130 160 820 825
Sample 4   116 220 405 410 550 735 835 705

You want to test the null hypothesis that the locations of all four samples are the same *against the general alternative that they are not all the same.*

4. You are studying a viral oncogene that induces anchorage-independent growth when expressed in fibroblasts. In order to map the functional domains within that oncogene, you construct a series of mutants and compare the abilities of the mutants to induce anchorage independent growth with that of the wild type gene. After co-transfecting the wild type or mutant oncogene with an antibiotic resistance marker into fibroblasts and selecting for antibiotic resistant cells, you plate 10^4 cells in agarose in each of a series of dishes. After allowing time for growth, you obtain the following numbers of colonies per dish.

wild type   120 310 440 413 500
mutant   48 15 120 15 23

Does this mutation inactivate the oncogene?

5. You have tested a particular chemical for its mutagenic activity in mammalian cells. In your experiment, you treated cells with various doses of the agent, allowed the cells to grow for a few generations and then plated 10^6 cells in the presence of 6-thioguanine to select for *hprt* mutants. After two weeks, you counted the mutant colonies. After doing the experiment several times, you obtained the following data:

Dose	Mutants/10^6 cells
0	2,0,5,3,1
10	3,9,8,8
20	17,41,12,5
40	80,79,44,56

Is the chemical mutagenic?

6. Analysis of Categorical Data

A variety of experiments generate data that are qualitative in nature such that the observations may be classified as belonging to one of two or more categories. Such data can be summarized conveniently as a table, generally referred to as a contingency table. We will often want to test hypotheses in which we are interested in the relationship between two or more different classification schemes.

6.1. The $1 \times c$ Table: Goodness of Fit Tests

The simplest contingency table is one dimensional. In this case, we may be interested in comparing the number of observations in each of the categories to those predicted by some predetermined model. As discussed in Chapter 4, our hypothesis may be simple, *i.e.*, the proportions in the categories are completely specified, or composite, *i.e.*, the proportions depend on one or more unknown parameters.

6.1.1. No unknown parameter to estimate.

We consider again, as in Example 4.2, the problem of deviation from Mendelian segregation. In this experiment, we observe particular numbers of animals of the three possible genotypes obtained in an intercross and want to test the hypothesis that the observed frequencies conform to the 1:2:1 proportions expected in the case that all three genotypes are recovered with similar efficiencies. More generally, we might classify n observations according to k categories and want to test the hypothesis that the observed n_i ($i=1 \dots k$) do not differ from that specified by a multinomial distribution in which all of the p_i are determined by the hypothesis. This "goodness of fit" test was first described by Pearson in 1900 and is based on the following statistic

$$X^2 = \sum_{i=1}^{k} \frac{(O_i - E_i)^2}{E_i}$$

When n is large, the observed frequencies will be normally distributed with a expected value of np_i and a variance of approximately the same magnitude. Thus, the value inside the summation can be seen to be approximately distributed as the square of a standardized normal variate. The sum of such squared normal values follows a χ^2 (Chi-square) distribution. Because it is sufficient to determine $(k - 1)$ of the p_i (they must add up to 1), the test statistic, X^2, follows a χ^2 distribution with $(k - 1)$ degrees of freedom. Although this distribution is difficult to compute, tables of the critical values for the distribution may be found in virtually any statistics text (see Appendix 3). Note that the χ^2 distribution is a good approximation only when n is relatively large. In practice the approximation is quite good when the expected frequencies are all greater than 5 and is still acceptable when the np_i are greater than 1.5.

Example 6.1 Deviation from Mendelian segregation.

We mate D/d animals and recover 1 D/D, 9 D/d, and 9 d/d offspring. If all of the progeny classes are recovered with equal efficiency, we expect proportions of 0.25, 0.5, and 0.25, respectively, giving expected numbers of 4.75, 9.5, and 4.75. We can compute the test statistic as

$$X^2 = \frac{(1-4.75)^2}{4.75} + \frac{(9-9.5)^2}{9.5} + \frac{(9-4.75)^2}{4.75}$$
$$= 6.8$$

Interpolating from the χ^2 distribution with 2 degrees of freedom, we obtain a significance level of $P<0.034$. You may wish to compare this analysis for general deviations from Mendelian segregation with the approach using the binomial distribution.

6.1.2. At least one unknown parameter to estimate.

A very common situation arises when the expected values are not completely determined by the hypothesis, but are functions of unknown parameters that must be estimated from the data. A typical genetic example is the testing of Hardy-Weinberg equilibrium.

Example 6.2 Deviation from Hardy-Weinberg equilibrium.

We draw a random sample from a population and find 20 *D/D*, 90 *D/d*, and 90 *d/d* individuals. The gene frequency for the D allele in the sample is $(40+90)/400 = 0.325$. So the expected numbers are 200×0.325^2, $400(0.325)(0.675)$, and 200×0.675^2.

We can compute the test statistic as

$$X^2 = \frac{(20-21.125)^2}{21.125} + \frac{(90-87.75)^2}{87.75} + \frac{(90-91.125)^2}{91.125}$$

$$= 0.132$$

In this case we refer to a χ^2 distribution with 1 degree of freedom. The *general rule* is that the degrees of freedom equal (the number of categories) $-$ 1 $-$ (the number of parameters estimated). In Example 6.1, no parameters were estimated and so we had 2 df. Here one parameter was estimated and we have only 1 df. Using the table in Appendix 3, we find that $P \sim 0.72$, and would conclude that the population conforms to HWE.

6.2. The 2 × 2 Table

Consider an experiment involving the analysis of categorical data, in which we make *n* observations and classify each observation according to whether or not it possesses two properties, A and B. After the experiment, we can tabulate the data as a 2 × 2 table, with the values n_{ij} representing the number of observations in the *i,j* cell and r_i and c_j the sum of the number of observations in row *i* and column *j*, respectively:

	B	~B	Total
A	n_{11}	n_{12}	r_1
~A	n_{21}	n_{22}	r_2
Total	c_1	c_2	n

6.2.1. *Four underlying sampling distributions.*

Four different experimental designs can give rise to the above 2×2 table depending on whether under repeated sampling n is variable, n is fixed, n and either the row or column totals are fixed, or n and both row and column totals are fixed. Consider the following examples.

Example 6.3
Model 0: Each cell entry is a random variable.

In this example each cell represents a Poisson variable, and, hence, the grand total is also a Poisson variable, *i.e.*, n is not fixed.

You sample numbers of accidents during 1999 on a particular road in Montana and classify them as to time of day and weather conditions. The results are:

	Day	Night
Dry	10	5
Wet	3	12

Since each entry is the realization of a Poisson random variable, the sum is also a random variable. However, if we condition our test on the observed sum, then the entries are multinomial random variables and the problem reduces to Example 6.4, below. This is a standard result and we will not prove it here.

Example 6.4
Model 1: Double dichotomy; row and column totals not fixed.

You are interested in testing the hypothesis that two RFLP markers, M_1 and M_2, are linked. You perform a backcross in which ($M_1^{D/B} M_2^{D/B}$) animals are mated to ($M_1^{B/B} M_2^{B/B}$) animals and analyze the genotypes of 30 progeny, *i.e.*, n is

---

fixed. You observe that 12 offspring are (B B / B B), 3 are (B D/B B), 5 are (D B/B B) and 10 are (D D / B B). If B^i indicates homozygosity at locus i and D^i indicates heterozygosity at locus i, we want to test the null hypothesis that

$$H_0: \ P[B^1B^2] = P[B^1] \times P[B^2]$$

against the one-sided alternative

$$H_1: \ P[B^1B^2] > P[B^1] \times P[B^2]$$

Example 6.5
Model 2: Test for homogeneity; row (or column) totals fixed.

You have developed a recombinant vaccine for a viral disease and want to test it for efficacy. You inoculate 15 animals with the vaccine and inject 15 animals with saline. All of the animals are then infected and the presence or absence of virus-induced disease is evaluated after 2 weeks. Among the control animals 12 develop the disease, while only 5 of the inoculated animals become ill. Using p_u and p_i to denote the probabilities of developing the disease for untreated and inoculated animals, respectively, we want to test the hypothesis

$$H_0: \ p_u = p_i$$

against the one-sided alternative

$$H_1: \ p_u > p_i$$

Example 6.6
Model 3: Both margins fixed.

It is difficult to define a good biological example for this case. You are studying a mutant that, when homozygous (*aa*), exhibits a fairly subtle phenotype that can be observed only on microscopic examination by someone who is highly trained. In order to test the ability of the person scoring for the phenotype, you assemble a collection of 30 animals, of which 17 are homozygous mutant and 13 are heterozygous (*Aa*) as determined by an independent method. You tell your scorer that all of the animals come from a backcross and ask that the animals be classified as homozygous mutant or heterozygous. Because the scorer is genetically trained, s/he will use the expected equal frequencies of the categories in making the assignments. Of the 17 mutant animals, the scorer assigns 12 correctly. Using the subscript conventions in the 2×2 table above, we want to test the hypothesis that our scorer does better at assigning the genotype than would be predicted by chance:

$$H_0: p_{11}/p_{1.} = p_{12}/p_{2.}$$
$$H_1: p_{11}/p_{1.} > p_{12}/p_{2.}$$

In spite of the differences in these experimental designs, each of the above examples yields the same 2×2 table. Quite remarkably, the same method provides a powerful test of each of the above hypotheses and the distribution of the test statistic is identical for all three null hypotheses. [Note that the same can not be said of the distribution under the alternative hypothesis, a matter we will revisit when discussing experimental design.] The method has its origin in considering the case with both margins fixed and is named for R. A. Fisher (1973).

6.2.2. Fisher's exact test: the hypergeometric distribution.

If all four of the marginal totals are fixed, the value of any one of the cells, *e.g.*, n_{11}, is sufficient to determine the entire table. Thus, the probability of obtaining any given 2×2 table can be obtained by considering the distribution of n_{11} conditional on n, r_1, and c_1. The appropriate probability is given by the hypergeometric distribution,

$$\Pr(n_{11}) = \frac{\binom{r_1}{n_{11}}\binom{r_2}{n_{21}}}{\binom{n}{c_1}} = \frac{r_1!\,r_2!\,c_1!\,c_2!}{n_{11}!\,n_{12}!\,n_{21}!\,n_{22}!\,n!}$$

For Example 6.6, we can define the following table

	True *Aa*	True *aa*	Total
Assign *Aa*	10	5	15
Assign *aa*	3	12	15
Total	13	17	30

Our scorer has made 15 *Aa* assignments, of which 10 are correct, and there are $\binom{15}{10}$ ways to do so. For each of these permutations, there are $\binom{15}{3}$ ways to incorrectly assign an *aa* genotype. Thus, the probability of making 10 correct *Aa* assignments is given by

$$p(n_{11} = 10) = \frac{\binom{15}{10}\binom{15}{3}}{\binom{30}{13}} = 0.0114$$

Similarly, we can compute the probabilities of making 11, 12, and 13 correct *Aa* assignments as 0.0012, 5.7×10^{-5}, and 8.8×10^{-7}, respectively. Thus, the probability of making 10 or more correct *Aa* assignments is approximately 0.0127, which is the significance level for our statistical test. The distribution for the test statistic is equivalent to that for the hypergeometric distribution, which arises in the case of sampling from a finite population without replacement. Note that this test is *exact* in the sense that we can directly compute the distribution of our test statistic (the value of n_{11}) under the null hypothesis.

The primary virtues of Fisher's exact test are that it makes optimum use of the available information and allows for a straightforward computation of the exact significance level. A disadvantage of this test is that computations by hand (*i.e.*, by pocket calculator) are cumbersome. To simplify computation of the *P*-value, organize the table such that c_1 is the smallest of the 4 marginal totals and n_{11} can increase in the direction specified by the one-sided alternative hypothesis. Then, the significance level is given by

$$\alpha = \sum_{x=n_{11}}^{x=\min(r_1,c_1)} f(x) \quad \text{where} \quad f(x) = \frac{\binom{r_1}{x}\binom{r_2}{c_1-x}}{\binom{n}{c_1}}$$

In the case that the row (or column) totals are equal, the hypergeometric distribution is symmetrical and the two-sided significance level can be obtained by simply doubling the value computed for the upper tail. When the row totals are not equal, the simplest way to compute the two-sided *P*-value is to compute the upper tail as above and compute the lower tail by summing the f(x) that are no larger than the value for f(n_{11}). This approach is used in the example below.

Example 6.7 Using Fisher's exact test for a two-sided alternative.

In a variation of the experiment described in Example 6.5, we are testing whether or not vaccination prevents or exacerbates a disease caused by infection with a particular agent. We vaccinate 10 animals and infect these animals along with 7 control animals. After two weeks, we find that 6 of the vaccinated animals and 2 of the control animals are healthy and the remaining animals suffer from the disease. We want to test the hypothesis

$$H_0: p_u = p_i$$
$$H_a: p_u \neq p_i$$

where p_u and p_i are the probabilities of illness in control and vaccinated animals, respectively. For this experiment, we obtain the following table with the distribution for all possible tables shown below. (Note that the table is rotated so that c_1 is the smallest marginal value.)

	Control	Vaccinated	Total
Ill	5	4	9
Healthy	2	6	8
Total	7	10	17

The observed table, in which $x=5$, has a probability of 0.181. There are 5 additional tables with probabilities that are less than or equal to that for the observed table. Summing these 6 possible outcomes, we obtain a significance level of 0.335.

x	$f(x)$
0	4×10^{-4}
1	0.013
2	0.104
3	0.302
4	0.363
5	0.181
6	0.034
7	0.002

6.2.3. An unconditional exact test.

Fisher's exact test is conditional on both the row and column totals (Model 3 above), but nonetheless provides an appropriate (albeit conservative) test in the case that only one of the margins (rows or columns) is fixed. Barnard (1947) described an exact, *unconditional* test for homogeneity (Model 2) that is more powerful than Fisher's conditional test under that model (Mártín Andres *et al.*, 2004).

Consider an experiment in which we compare two groups (*e.g.*, treated and control), each with a number of observations fixed by design, for the proportion of subjects exhibiting some response. We can tabulate our results in the familiar 2 × 2 table

	Responder	Non-responder	Total
Treatment	x_1	$r_1 - x_1$	r_1
Control	x_2	$r_2 - x_2$	r_2
Total	$(x_1 + x_2)$	$n - x_1 - x_2$	n

We want to test the hypothesis that the probability of responding in the treatment group, p_1, is the same as that in the control group, p_2,

$$H_0: p_1 = p_2$$

against, for example, the one-sided alternative

$$H_1: p_1 > p_2$$

Here we suppose that, under the null hypothesis, the common probability of responding for the two groups is p. Then, the probability of obtaining our observed table, T_o, is the product of two binomials:

$$P(T_o \mid p) = \binom{r_1}{x_1}\binom{r_2}{x_2} p^{x_1+x_2}(1-p)^{n-x_1-x_2}$$

To obtain the P-value for our test, we need to consider some critical region (CR) that contains all of the tables that represent an outcome at least as extreme as our observed table. Then, the significance level $\alpha(p)$ can be obtained by summing the above probabilities over all of the tables in the CR.

$$\alpha(p) = \sum_{CR} \binom{r_1}{x_1}\binom{r_2}{x_2} p^{x_1+x_2}(1-p)^{n-x_1-x_2}$$

Of course, the value of p under the null hypothesis is unknown; it is a nuisance parameter. As discussed by Barnard, the significance level, α^*, can be determined by finding the value of p that maximizes the above equation, that is,

$$\alpha^* = \max_{0<p<1} \alpha(p)$$

All that remains is to define the critical region for the test. In Barnard's original paper, the CR is built up iteratively following a few simple rules.

Start with the most extreme possible outcome, where $x_1=0$ and $x_2=r_2$, and compute α^*. The next possible table is added to the CR from among those that satisfy the rule of convexity, *i.e.*, the newly added table must be immediately adjacent to the CR. The table that is added is the one that increases α^* by the smallest amount (the rule of minimum). In the case of a two-sided test, a symmetry rule is applied. When a table is added to the CR, the corresponding table from the opposite tail is added simultaneously. This algorithm for building the CR is referred to in Barnard's paper as the CSM method, and it is repeated until the observed table is the last table added to the critical region.

The CSM method described by Barnard is computationally very demanding, because the maximization step to obtain α^* must be performed many times to build up the critical region. The 1947 paper includes tables for the P-values for experiments in which r_1 and r_2 are (7,7), (6,8), and (5,9), which must have taken many weeks to compute by hand. Various less computationally demanding approaches to defining the CR have been proposed based on using an alternative statistic, $S(T)$, and including all tables for which $S(T)$ is more extreme than that for the observed table. Two common choices for $S(T)$ include the Chi-square test (see section 6.2.4) and Fisher's exact test. The latter has been shown to be nearly as powerful as the CSM method over a wide range of r_1/r_2 (Martín Andrés and Silva Mato, 1994).

Example 6.8

We are interested in comparing the incidence of spontaneous liver tumors in two inbred mouse strains. Male mice of each strain are analyzed at 15 months of age for the presence or absence of liver cancer to obtain the following results

	Tumor	Tumor-free	Total
Strain 1	1	20	21
Strain 2	5	12	17
Total	6	32	38

We want to test the null hypothesis that tumor incidence is the same for the two strains, $p_1=p_2$, against the two-sided alternative that they are different, $p_1 \neq p_2$.

The CR is built up using the CSM method to obtain the following (1 indicates the table is included and the observed table is shaded)

	0	1	2	3	4	5	6	7	8	9	10	11	12	13	14	15	16	17	18	19	20	21
17	1	1	1	1	1	1	1	1	1	1	1	1	1	1	1	1	1	0	0	0	0	0
16	1	1	1	1	1	1	1	1	1	1	1	1	1	1	1	0	0	0	0	0	0	0
15	1	1	1	1	1	1	1	1	1	1	1	1	1	0	0	0	0	0	0	0	0	0
14	1	1	1	1	1	1	1	1	1	1	1	0	0	0	0	0	0	0	0	0	0	1
13	1	1	1	1	1	1	1	1	1	1	0	0	0	0	0	0	0	0	0	0	0	1
12	1	1	1	1	1	1	1	1	0	0	0	0	0	0	0	0	0	0	0	0	1	1
11	1	1	1	1	1	1	1	0	0	0	0	0	0	0	0	0	0	0	0	0	1	1
10	1	1	1	1	1	1	0	0	0	0	0	0	0	0	0	0	0	0	0	1	1	1
9	1	1	1	1	1	0	0	0	0	0	0	0	0	0	0	0	0	0	1	1	1	1
8	1	1	1	1	0	0	0	0	0	0	0	0	0	0	0	0	0	1	1	1	1	1
7	1	1	1	0	0	0	0	0	0	0	0	0	0	0	0	0	1	1	1	1	1	1
6	1	1	0	0	0	0	0	0	0	0	0	0	0	0	0	1	1	1	1	1	1	1
5	1	**1**	0	0	0	0	0	0	0	0	0	0	0	0	1	1	1	1	1	1	1	1
4	1	0	0	0	0	0	0	0	0	0	0	0	1	1	1	1	1	1	1	1	1	1
3	1	0	0	0	0	0	0	0	0	0	1	1	1	1	1	1	1	1	1	1	1	1
2	0	0	0	0	0	0	0	0	1	1	1	1	1	1	1	1	1	1	1	1	1	1
1	0	0	0	0	0	0	0	1	1	1	1	1	1	1	1	1	1	1	1	1	1	1
0	0	0	0	0	0	1	1	1	1	1	1	1	1	1	1	1	1	1	1	1	1	1

Maximizing $\alpha(p)$ we obtain

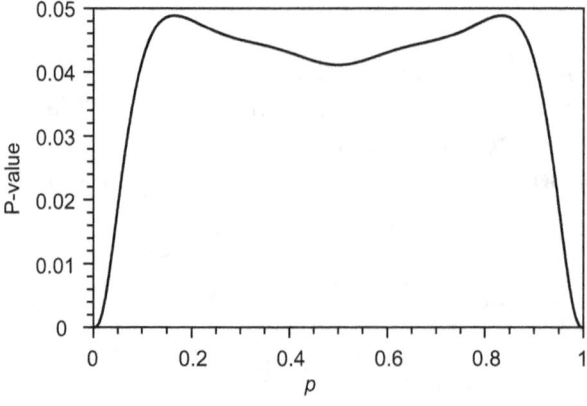

and find that the maximum occurs at $p = 0.166$, to give our two-sided P-value of 0.049. Note that Fisher's exact test would give a two-sided P-value of 0.071.

6.2.4. The Chi-square test.

The Chi-square test is the classical test for independence in a 2×2 table (Model 1), in which only n, the total number of observations, is fixed. This test may also be applied to 2×2 tables under the other models in which the rows and/or column totals are fixed. The test statistic is:

$$X^2 = \sum \frac{(O_{ij} - E_{ij})^2}{E_{ij}} = \frac{n(n_{11}n_{22} - n_{12}n_{21})^2}{r_1 r_2 c_1 c_2}$$

This test statistic may be referred to the χ^2 (Chi-square) distribution with 1 df (in the case of the two-sided alternative), or by making use of the fact that X is distributed as a standard normal distribution with mean 0 and variance 1. The latter may be used to test against one- or two-sided alternatives to the null hypothesis of equal success probabilities for the two treatments defined by the row categories.

6.2.5. Comparison of tests for 2 × 2 tables.

The three tests discussed above are motivated by three different experimental models, depending on whether neither, either, or both the row and/or column totals are fixed by design. The tests also range in computational difficulty from trivial (Chi-square) to modest (Fisher's exact test) to substantial (Barnard's exact test). Which test should you use for any give experimental context?

The derivation of Fisher's exact test was based on a model in which both the row and column sums are fixed in advance, a relatively uncommon experimental design. You will more often analyze data for experiments in which either n randomly chosen individuals are classified according to the row and column categories (neither r_i nor c_j fixed) or predetermined numbers of individuals are drawn at random from two or more populations and classified according to characteristic or response (either r_i or c_j fixed). For these two experimental designs, the P-value calculated using Fisher's exact test is conditional on the row and column totals. As discussed by Conover (1999), if the conditional P-value under H_0 is α, then the unconditional probability under H_0 is always less than or equal to α. Thus, the exact test remains valid for the cases in which the row and/or column totals are random variables. However, in these cases, Fisher's exact test tends to be conservative, yielding a larger P-value than the true α. For example, Storer and Kim (1990) found that the power of Fisher's exact test is 10-20% lower than that for the approximate (X or X^2) test when moderate sample sizes (more than 20 per group) are tested for a difference in proportions. Note, however, that the latter, approximate test statistics converge to normal or χ^2 distributions as $n \rightarrow \infty$. The quality of these approximations also depends on the expected numbers of observations per cell, and is relatively poor when there are cell counts smaller than 5. The estimated P-value may be larger or smaller than the true value of α, *i.e.*, Chi-square tests may be too conservative *or* too liberal when the sample size or cell counts are small.

For a model in which either the row or column totals are fixed, Barnard's exact test provides a reasonable alternative. Barnard's exact test was used rarely in the decades after its publication because the maximization step is computationally very demanding when compared to Fisher's exact test. However, Barnard's test is more powerful than Fisher's for the case of one fixed margin when the marginal totals are small, largely because the highly discrete nature of Fisher's exact test provides fewer possibilities in terms of the computed P-value (Martín Andrés and Silva Mato, 1994; Martín Andrés *et al.*, 2004). The controversy over which of the two exact tests should be used has continued since the initial publication by Barnard (Kempthorne, 1979). One source of contention is the appropriateness of the binomial model. Consider an experiment in which you want to compare the prevalence of some phenotype in two groups of mice of different genotype. One can readily envision each group as having been drawn at random from a notionally infinite population of mice representing that genotype, leading to a binomial model in which only the group sizes are fixed, which would make Barnard's exact test most appropriate.

On the other hand, consider the following clinical trial. You want to compare the effectiveness of a standard treatment regimen with one in which patients are treated with an augmented version that includes an additional drug. You identify the next 80 patients that come into the clinic with the disease of interest and randomly assign them to the two treatments in equal numbers. It may reasonably be argued that these 80 patients do not represent a random sample of all potential patients and that, under the null hypothesis of no difference between treatments, the total number of responders is fixed. In that case, both the row and column totals should be viewed as fixed and Fisher's exact test would be most appropriate.

Thus, there is no simple answer to the question posed above for experiments in which the row and/or column totals are not fixed. Our advice is to use one of the exact tests when sample sizes are small (*e.g.*, $r_i \leq$ 50) or when one or more of the cells contain fewer than 5 observations. Using an exact test for these cases insures that the true value of α is *no larger than* the calculated *P*-value. When the experiment involves fixed group sizes, you should choose between Fisher's and Barnard's exact test based on your view of the appropriateness of the binomial model. In any event, you should decide which test to use before you begin the analysis: It is never appropriate to shop among statistical tests for the *P*-value you find most desirable.

6.3. Paired data and structural zeros

6.3.1. McNemar's test for analysis of paired data.

For all of the cases described above, the *n* observations in the 2×2 table are independent. Example 6.7 represents a frequently encountered experimental approach. We assign at random members of a population to two distinct groups (vaccinated and control) and are interested in testing the null hypothesis that the probability of some outcome (*e.g.*, illness) is the same for the two groups. An alternative experimental design, in which each sample consists of a pair of observations, may be more appropriate when "uninteresting" sources of variation, in addition to the variable represented by our experimental groups, may contribute to the outcome we observe.

Consider the problem of testing the hypothesis that the incidence of a disease is greater among individuals with a particular genotype at a specific locus when compared with other members of the population. We could test that hypothesis in a prospective study by identifying a sufficient number of members of each group and monitoring them for the development of the disease over some fixed period of time. At the end of the study, our data would consist of the familiar 2×2 table, which may be analyzed using Fisher's exact test:

	Diseased	Healthy	Total
Genotype 1	n_{11}	n_{12}	r_1
Not Genotype 1	n_{21}	n_{22}	r_2
Total	c_1	c_2	n

This experimental design is expensive if the disease we are studying is relatively infrequent in both groups, is also influenced by many factors other than genotype, or develops after a long and variable period of time. An alternative strategy is to test the hypothesis in a retrospective, case-control study, in which we identify a number of individuals suffering from the disease (cases), choose for each an individual (control) that is similar to our case from a disease-free population, and determine the genotypes for both individuals in each paired sample. Four outcomes are possible for each (case, control) pair, where 1 indicates that the individual has Genotype 1: (1,1), (1,0), (0,1), (0,0). We could organize the data as shown in the table below.

Controls

Cases		Gen. 1	Not Gen. 1	Total
	Gen. 1	a	b	$(a+b)$
	Not Gen. 1	c	d	$(c+d)$
	Total	$(a+c)$	$(b+d)$	n

This problem can be viewed as a variation on the Sign test alluded to in Problem 7 of Section 2.5. The a and d concordant pairs (both case and control have the same genotype classification) represent tied values and can be discarded from the analysis. Under the null hypothesis that the prevalences of Genotype 1 among the cases and controls are equal, the two types of discordant pairs [events (1,0) and (0,1)] will each occur with a probability of 0.5. Thus, we can use the binomial distribution with parameters $p=0.5$ and $N=b+c$ to test our hypothesis (McNemar, 1947). For the one-sided alternative that (1,0) pairs are more frequent than (0,1) pairs, the exact P-value can be computed from:

$$P_1 = \sum_{x=b}^{b+c} \binom{b+c}{x} 0.5^{b+c}$$

The P-value for the two-sided alternative may be obtained by adding to P_1 the value for the lower tail of the binomial distribution, *i.e.*, summing the values for $x=0$ to $x=c$. Results for experiments of this type are often reported in terms of the odds ratio, which is simply b/c.

6.3.2. The structural zero.

All 2×2 tables are not necessarily contingency tables. Consider the hypothetical example below:

Secondary Infection

		Yes	No
Primary Infection	Yes	20	60
	No	0	60

One of the four cells is zero, not because we just happened to pick up a zero through random fluctuation, but because one cannot have a secondary infection without first having had a primary infection; the zero is said to be a structural zero. The hypothesis to be tested is that primary and secondary infections are equal and independent.

Let p=Pr(of infection). Then under the null hypothesis, the likelihood is

$$L = (p^2)^A (p(1-p))^B (1-p)^C \quad \text{where } A=20, B=60, \text{ and } C=60.$$

The maximum likelihood estimator of p is

$$\hat{p} = \frac{2A+B}{2A+2B+C}$$

with a variance of $V=p(1-p)/[n(1+p)]$. For our data $\hat{p} = \dfrac{5}{11}$ and so the expected values of A, B, and C are 28.93, 34.71, and 76.36, respectively. We may now apply the Chi-square goodness of fit test for which we have three classes and one parameter estimated, yielding 1 df: $X^2 = 24.69$.

Clearly, first and second infections are either not equal or not independent; *e.g.*, there are far too many in the "Yes, No" cell.

6.3.3. Another goodness of fit test masquerading as a 2 ×2 contingency table.

Here is one more example of a 2×2 table which is actually a goodness of fit problem with 3 degrees of freedom. The data are of one of Mendel's original two-factor crosses (F_2):

	Yellow	Green	Total
Round	315	108	423
Wrinkled	101	32	133
Total	416	140	556

In this case there are no parameters to estimate: We expect from Mendel's theory that the cell entries should be in a 9:3:3:1 ratio, and that the two marginals (row and column totals) should each be in a 3:1 ratio. Testing for the 9:3:3:1 ratio, the total $X^2=0.47$ with 3 df. The row and column totals yield Chi-squares of 0.3453 and 0.0096, respectively, each with 1 df. The difference 0.47 - 0.3453 - 0.0096 = 0.115 with 1 df is a pure test of linkage. We see that the 3 df Chi-square test may be partitioned into three individual tests, each with 1 df. We will discuss the partitioning of contingency tables more generally later in this chapter.

6.4. The $r \times c$ Table

We now extend our analysis of contingency tables to the case of any arbitrary number of rows and columns. Our data consist of n observations classified according to r row categories and c column categories as in the table below.

n_{11}	n_{12}	$\cdots$	n_{1c}	r_1
n_{21}	n_{22}	$\cdots$	n_{2c}	r_2
$\vdots$	$\vdots$	$\vdots$	$\vdots$	$\vdots$
n_{r1}	n_{r2}	$\cdots$	n_{rc}	r_r
c_1	c_2	$\cdots$	c_c	n

6.4.1. The exact test: Extended hypergeometric distribution.

For an $r \times c$ table, the generalization of the hypergeometric exact probability distribution is given by

$$\Pr(\{n_{ij}\} \,|\, \{c_i, r_j\}) = \frac{\prod (c_i!) \prod (r_j!)}{n! \prod (n_{ij}!)}$$

This distribution is no longer one-dimensional and how to order the tables is not immediately apparent. Consider the example below.

Example 6.9 Exact Analysis of a 3 × 2 table.

We are interested in the effects of pregnancy on the induction of mammary tumors in rats. Animals with a prior history of 0, 1, or more than 1 pregnancy are treated with a carcinogen at 6 months of age and analyzed for the presence of mammary tumors at 14 months of age. We obtain the following

	Tumor-bearing	Tumor-free	Total
Nulliparous	2	2	4
Uniparous	3	2	5
Multiparous	0	6	6
Total	5	10	15

There are exactly 20 tables that correspond to the fixed row and column totals; they are shown below. The numbers directly above each table are the value of the Chi-square test statistic for that table and its exact probability (out of 3003).

11.25
6

0	4
0	5
5	1

5.625
60

1	3
0	5
4	2

3.75
120

2	2
0	5
3	3

5.625
60

3	1
0	5
2	4

11.25
6

4	0
0	5
1	5

5.4
75

0	4
1	4
4	2

1.275
400

1	3
1	4
3	3

0.90
450

2	2
1	4
2	4

4.225
120

3	1
1	4
1	5

11.4
5

4	0
1	4
0	6

2.25
200

0	4
2	3
3	3

0.225
600

1	3
2	3
2	4

1.35
360

2	2
2	3
1	5

6.225
40

3	1
2	3
0	6

3.6
150

0	4
3	2
2	4

2.475
240

1	3
3	2
1	5

5.10
60

2	**2**
3	**2**
0	**6**

(**bold** is observed table)

7.65
30

0	4
4	1
1	5

8.025
20

1	3
4	1
0	6

15.00
1

0	4
5	0
0	6

Now, how might we arrange these tables? At least two methods suggest themselves; by the size of the Chi-square test statistic, or by their exact probabilities. Let us look at the result.

Exact Pr	1	5	6^2	20	30	40	60^3	75
Chi-square	15.00	11.4	11.25	8.025	7.65	6.225	5.10	5.4
							5.625^2	

Exact Pr	120^2	150	200	240	360	400	450	600
Chi-square	4.275	3.6	2.85	2.475	1.35	1.275	0.9	0.225
	3.75							

We see that the two methods lead generally to the same ordering, but not quite. If we order the tables by Chi-square and sum up probabilities of all those tables with Chi-square values at least as large as the table we observed yields 0.1209, whereas if we order by exact probabilities, we get 0.096. Usually, the ordering criterion will make little difference, but the fact that they need not be exactly the same is a complication one must be aware of. Here, had we been testing at the 10% level, it would have made a difference.

6.4.2. The Chi-square test.

Under the null hypothesis that the row and column classifications are independent, we can determine the expected proportion for each cell from the fixed row and column totals as

$$p_{ij} = \frac{r_i c_j}{n^2}$$

As in the case of the 2×2 table, we may use the Chi-square test statistic,

$$X^2 = \sum \frac{(O_{ij} - E_{ij})^2}{E_{ij}} = \sum_{i=1}^{r} \sum_{j=1}^{c} \frac{(n_{ij} - np_{ij})^2}{np_{ij}}$$

This statistic follows a χ^2 distribution with

$$(rc\text{-}1)\text{-}(r\text{-}1)\text{-}(c\text{-}1) = (r\text{-}1)(c\text{-}1)$$

degrees of freedom. Note, again, we are using the general principle that the number of degrees of freedom is df = (number of cells) – 1 – (number of parameters estimated).

Example 6.10 Analysis of a 3 × 2 table.

We repeat Example 6.9 with realistic numbers. We are interested in the effects of pregnancy on the induction of mammary tumors in rats. Animals with a prior history of 0, 1, or more than 1 pregnancy are treated with a carcinogen at 6 months of age and analyzed for the presence of mammary tumors at 14 months of age. We obtain the following data (with expected values in parentheses)

	Tumor-bearing	Tumor-free	Total
Nulliparous	3 (8.32)	14 (8.68)	17
Uniparous	8 (7.83)	8 (8.17)	16
Multiparous	12 (6.85)	2 (7.14)	14
Total	23	24	47

Summing the statistic over the 6 cells, we obtain a value of 14.25. Using the χ^2 distribution with (3-1) (2-1) = 2 degrees of freedom, our significance level is $P<0.001$ and we would reject the hypothesis that susceptibility to mammary carcinogenesis is independent of parity.

6.4.3. An equivalent likelihood ratio test.

In the discussion above, we were interested in testing the hypothesis that the row and column classifications for the n observations in the $r \times c$ table are independent. Consider an alternative experimental design. We have obtained r independent samples, each consisting of r_i observations, corresponding to different treatment groups. For each treatment, we classify the observations according to c mutually exclusive categories. We want to test the null hypothesis

$$H_0: p_{1j} = p_{2j} = \ldots = p_{rj} \text{ for all } j$$

against the general alternative that at least one pair of success probabilities is different.

Under the null hypothesis, the maximum likelihood estimates (see section 3.2) for the column probabilities are $\hat{p}_j = c_j / n$, while the unrestricted maximum likelihood estimates are $\hat{p}_{ij} = n_{ij} / r_i$.

Thus, we can define the likelihood ratio statistic as

$$G^2 = 2\sum_{i=1}^{r}\sum_{j=1}^{c} n_{ij} \times \ln\left(\frac{n \times n_{ij}}{r_i c_j}\right)$$

As with the Chi-square test, the likelihood ratio statistic approximately follows a χ^2 distribution with $(r-1)(c-1)$ degrees of freedom. In general, the Chi-square and likelihood ratio tests will give similar results and lead to the same conclusions. For the parity example given above, the value of G^2 is 15.63 (compared with 14.25 for X^2), yielding a P-value of 4×10^{-4}. The χ^2 approximation for both X^2 and G^2 improves with increasing sample size and expected cell counts, but the approximation is closer for the former statistic when some of the expected cell counts are smaller than 5.

6.4.4. Partitioning r × c tables.

A very useful property of Chi-square statistics is their additivity for multiple, independent tests. That is, the sum of two independent Chi-square statistics with degrees of freedom d_1 and d_2, respectively, also follows a χ^2 distribution with $d_1 + d_2$ degrees of freedom. This property allows us to partition an $r \times c$ table into $(r-1)(c-1)$ tests (each a 2×2 table) with 1 degree of freedom.

To partition a table, order the rows and columns in a way that allows you to make the desired comparisons. Start at the upper left corner of the table, and compute X^2 or G^2 for the resulting 2×2 table. For each remaining cell in the $(r-1) \times (c-1)$ portion at the lower-right of the original table, form a new 2×2 table with the value in the selected cell placed as n_{22} and the rest of the table filled in by summing the values upward and/or to the left, as appropriate. For example, a 3×4 table can be partitioned into 6 tests, with n_{22} containing the cells labeled 6, 7, 8, 10, 11, or 12, as indicated below.

$$1 \quad 2 \quad 3 \quad 4$$
$$5 \quad 6 \quad 7 \quad 8$$
$$9 \quad 10 \quad 11 \quad 12$$

The 2×2 table for cell 11 is

$$(1+2+5+6) \quad (3+7)$$
$$(9+10) \qquad 11$$

Adding together the values of G^2 for all of the partitions should equal (exactly, outside of rounding) the value of G^2 for the table as a whole, while the sum of the X^2 values for the partitions will only approximate the value of X^2 for the original table.

Example 6.11

In a study of the relation between the ABO blood groups and certain diseases, a large sample of patients and controls was collected. (The numbers of AB individuals were so small they are not shown).

Blood type	Controls	Peptic Ulcer	Gastric Cancer
A	2625	679	416
B	570	134	84
O	2892	983	383

Analyzing the table as a whole, we obtain a likelihood ratio statistic of $G^2 = 40.6$. Using the χ^2 distribution with 4 degrees of freedom, the resulting P-value is 3×10^{-8}, allowing us to conclude that gastric disease is strongly associated with blood type. Our four partitions are

2625 679 $G^2 = 0.84, P = 0.36$
 570 134

3195 813 $G^2 = 28.96, P = 7\times10^{-8}$

2892 983

3304 416 $G^2 = 0.18$, $P = 0.67$
704 84

4008 500 $G^2 = 10.66$, $P = 0.001$
3875 383

From our partitioned analysis, we could conclude that having blood type O is strongly associated with peptic ulcers and, to a lesser extent, gastric cancer.

Our example of partitioning an $r \times c$ table follows a set of more general rules:

1. The df of the sub-tables must sum to the df of the original table.

2. Each cell count in the original table must be a cell count in one and only one sub-table.

3. Each marginal total of the original table must be a marginal total for one and only one sub-table.

Notice that under these more general rules, the sub-tables need not be 2×2 tables.

6.5. Ordered Categories

In the statistical tests we discussed above, the order within the rows or categories had no effect on our analysis. However, for some experiments, the rows, columns, or both sets of categories may follow a natural order (*e.g.*, age, dose of a test substance, the three genotypes in an intercross). Taking that ordering into account can provide us with a more powerful statistical test of particular hypotheses.

6.5.1. Ordered rows or columns: Cochran-Armitage test.

Consider the problem of testing for a trend in a dichotomous response for a data set consisting of r ordered rows. Below, we follow the treatment provided by Agresti (2002). For row i, let $\pi_{1|i}$ be the true probability of response 1, and $p_{1|i}$ be the observed proportion. Also let x_i denote some score assigned to the ith row. Then for a strictly linear trend, we would have

$$\pi_{1|i} = a + bx_i$$

and the least squares prediction equation

$$\hat{\pi}_{1|i} = p_{+1} + b(x_i - \bar{x}), \text{ where}$$

$$\bar{x} = \frac{\sum n_{i+} x_i}{n} \text{ and } b = \frac{\sum n_{i+}(p_{1|i} - p_{+1})(x_i - \bar{x})}{\sum n_{i+}(x_i - \bar{x})^2}$$

In the above formulas, n_{i+} is the total for row i and p_{+1} is the sum over column 1 divided by the total number of observations. This result is straightforward linear regression theory (see Chapter 8).

The Cochran-Armitage test (Cochran, 1954; Armitage, 1955) provides a way to partition the total Chi-square into two parts: the first, X^2 (trend), has 1 df and tests for a linear trend in the row proportions; the second, X^2 (model), has r-2 df (r is the number of rows) and tests the goodness of fit of the model, itself.

$$X^2(trend) = \left(\frac{b^2}{p_{+1}p_{+2}}\right)\sum n_{i+}(x_i - \bar{x})^2$$

$$X^2(model) = \left(\frac{1}{p_{+1}p_{+2}}\right)\sum n_{i+}(p_{1|i} - \hat{\pi}_{1|i})^2$$

Example 6.12 Trend in ordered rows.

The data below were presented by a graduate student interested in testing if there is a trend over time in the use of birth control. We have a 10 × 2 contingency table; but what is special is that the rows are ordered (ordinal, rather than nominal). Ignoring the ordering for a moment we get a regular contingency table Chi-square test statistic of 85.07 with

9 df. Clearly, year and use of birth controls are not independent. But, is there any consistent trend?

Year	Birth Control Use at Time of Screen		Total Women
	Do Not Use	Use	
1978	158 (91.9%)	14 (8.1%)	172
1981	108 (85%)	19 (15%)	127
1984	103 (85.8%)	17 (14.2%)	120
1987	71 (72.4%)	27 (27.6%)	98
1990	63 (76.9%)	19 (23.1%)	82
1995	65 (64.4%)	36 (35.6%)	101
1996	44 (62.9%)	26 (37.1%)	70
1997	29 (70.7%)	12 (29.3%)	41
1998	24 (68.6%)	11 (31.4%)	35
1999	12 (35.3%)	22 (64.7%)	34
Total	677 (76.9%)	203 (23.1%)	880

For our data, above, we chose, as the x_i the years, themselves, $(78, 81, 84, ...)$. The value of p_{+1} is 677/880 or 0.769. We find

b= -0.0162806 and $\bar{x} = 87.2466$ and

$$X^2 \ (trend) = 68.16 \text{ with 1 df}$$

$$X^2 \ (model) = 16.91 \text{ with 8 df.}$$

These values sum to the total X^2 already calculated. There is certainly a trend, but the model doesn't really fit very well, likely because the trend is not really linear.

6.5.2. Ordered rows and columns: Jonckheere-Terpstra test.

As shown in the example below, you can apply the Jonckheere-Terpstra test (section 5.4.2) to a contingency table that has both rows and columns ordered.

Example 6.13 Ordered rows and columns

Consider the following experiment in which wild-type, heterozygous, and homozygous mutant mice are compared for
the severity of motor defect:

Genotype	Motor defect		
	None	Mild	Severe
AA	10	2	0
Aa	5	8	2
aa	3	7	8

This is a contingency table with both rows (number of mutant alleles) and columns (severity of defect) naturally ordered, and $n=45$.

Applying the Jonckheere-Terpstra test to these data (taking
into account the ties, of course), we get U= 507.5 with E(U)=
333 and V(U)=1985.8. So the normal test statistic is Z= 3.92,
which corresponds to P=0.0001, for a two-sided test.

6.6. Higher Dimensional Tables

Although our examples so far have consisted of one or two dimensional contingency tables, the approximate methods, based on X^2 and G^2,
may be applied readily to data in higher dimensions. In the discussion below, we analyze a three dimensional table and illustrate an inherent pitfall
in the analysis of contingency tables.

6.6.1. The 2 × 2 × 2 table and Simpson's paradox.

Consider the following data on smoking and cancer reported by an
imaginary tobacco company in the 1960's.

	Cancer	No Cancer
Non-Smokers	190 (0.118)	1419
Smokers	182 (0.103)	1489

It appears from the table that smokers have slightly lower cancer rates that non-smokers. The result is not significant, but there is certainly no evidence in the data, as presented, of a risk from smoking.

But now, let us look at the original data which were actually in the form of a $2 \times 2 \times 2$ table in which males and females are counted separately.

Women	Cancer	No Cancer	Men	Cancer	No Cancer
Non-Smokers	188 (0.12)	1318	Non-Smokers	2 (0.02)	101
Smokers	112 (0.17)	522	Smokers	70 (0.06)	967

When the data are subdivided into males and females we find that in both sexes there is a higher rate of cancer among smokers (in females it is even statistically significant). At face value, it appears that smoking is bad for males and bad for females, but good for people in general! Obviously collapsing the two tables into one results in a totally misleading impression. Fortunately, this sort of extreme result of collapsing of a higher dimensional table into a smaller dimensional one does not happen often, but it is always a possibility. *The sobering fact to remember is that all contingency tables are collapsed tables*—collapsed over all those categories you did not think of taking into account or were unable to measure.

6.6.2. A Plethora of Hypotheses

Multidimensional tables, like the one above, lead to many more hypotheses than just the question of independence versus non-independence; various kinds of conditional independences emerge. Using the hypothetical smoking data as an example, we show a more detailed analysis of these data.

Smoking and Cancer Example
(V=Smoking status, S=sex, C=Cancer status)

Model	G^2	df	P value	df	Expected values
1. (S)(V)(C)	1315.64	4	$<10^{-3}$	$IJK-I-J-K+2$	$n_{i..}n_{.j.}n_{..k}/n^2$
2. (VC)(S)	1267.85	3	$<10^{-3}$	$(I-1)(JK-1)$	$n_{i..}n_{.jk}/n$
3. (SC)(V)	1314.96	3	$<10^{-3}$	$(J-1)(IK-1)$	$n_{.j.}n_{i.k}/n$
4. (SV)(C)	62.20	3	$<10^{-3}$	$(K-1)(IJ-1)$	$n_{..k}n_{ij.}/n$
5. (SC)(VC)	1267.16	2	$<10^{-3}$	$K(I-1)(J-1)$	$n_{i.k}n_{.jk}/n_{..k}$
6. (SC)(SV)	61.52	2	$<10^{-3}$	$I(J-1)(K-1)$	$n_{ij.}n_{i.k}/n_{i..}$
7. (VC)(SV)	14.41	2	0.001	$J(I-1)(K-1)$	$n_{ij.}n_{.jk}/n_{.j.}$
8. (SC)(VC)(SV)	1.88	1	0.18	$(I-1)(J-1)(K-1)$	by iteration (see Agresti 2002, chapter 6.)

The meanings of the eight hypotheses are as follows:

1. Sex, smoking status, and cancer state are mutually independent.
2. Sex is jointly independent of smoking and cancer.
3. Smoking is jointly independent of sex and cancer.
4. Cancer is jointly independent of sex and smoking.
5. Sex and smoking are independent given cancer.
6. Cancer and smoking are independent given sex.
7. Cancer and sex are independent given smoking.
8. No pair is even conditionally independent.

In our data, only the last hypothesis fits the data, so collapsing the $2 \times 2 \times 2$ table into a 2×2 table was definitely unwarranted.

6.6.3. Loglinear Models

There is a extensive literature on the analysis of multidimensional tables using what are called "loglinear models." Essentially, these models treat statistical dependencies as interactions by writing the expected values in terms of logs. We will not deal with loglinear models in this book, but see Agresti (2002) for a detailed discussion of this very important method of analysis.

6.7. Sample Problems

1. Two inbred mouse strains, C57BL and RFM, are compared for their risk for developing spontaneous lymphomas. Forty male animals of each strain are housed under identical conditions and allowed to live out their normal lifespan, which averaged 20 months for both strains. The incidences of lymphoma were 3/40 for C57BL mice and 8/40 for RFM mice. Do these two strains differ in their risk for lymphoma development?

2. Reanalyze the data in Example 6.8 using the X^2-test. Does the significance level differ than that obtained using Fisher's exact test? What might account for this difference?

3. The X^2 test of fit can be used to test composite hypotheses related to, for example, the form of the distribution. You are studying tumor development in the lung and for a particular group of animals, you observe the data below:

Number of Tumors	0	1	2	3	4	5
Number of Mice	13	7	3	1	1	1

You want to test the hypothesis that the tumor multiplicity is distributed according to a Poisson distribution. To perform the test, estimate the Poisson parameter and use it to determine the expected values for the distribution (pool the last 3 categories so that the expected numbers are reasonable). The number of degrees of freedom should be reduced by 1 to account for the fact that you have estimated one of the parameters for the distribution.

4. You are comparing four independent mutant alleles for their abilities to cause a developmental defect that is scored as absent, moderate, or severe. In the table below, is the expression of the defect independent of the allele?

	Absent	Moderate	Severe
allele 1	10	4	4
allele 2	5	8	2
allele 3	6	2	1
allele 4	3	7	8

5. The following are real data from Radelet and Pierce (1991) and quoted in Agresti (2007). The study was initiated to examine the effect of race on whether individuals convicted of homicide receive the death penalty or not. The data are of 674 subjects convicted of homicide in 20 Florida counties during 1976-1987.

		Death Penalty	
		Yes	No
Race of	White	53	430
Defendant	Black	15	176

The 2×2 table above is actually a summarization of the complete data. The complete data were in the form of the 2×2×2 table shown below:

		Victim White			Victim Black	
		Death Penalty			Death Penalty	
		Yes	No		Yes	No
Race of	White	53	414	White	0	16
Defendant	Black	11	37	Black	4	139

Examine these tables carefully. What is so strange about these data? How do you explain it? How would you analyze such data?

6. Different types of 2 × 2 tables. Analyze each of the tables given below. Although a minimum of information is provided, think about how the data were collected. How many degrees of freedom are appropriate for each example?

a. Tea Tasting Lady

		guess		
		SM	MS	
set	SM	4	11	15
	MS	11	14	25
		15	25	40

b. Traffic accidents

	Dry	Wet	
Day	10	20	30
Night	14	32	46
	24	52	76

c. Pneumonia in calves

		2° infection		
		Y	N	
1°	Y	30	63	93
inf	N	0	63	63
		30	126	156

d. Testing a Drug

	live	die	
Trt.	16	4	20
Con.	8	12	20
	24	16	40

e. Population Sample

		Hair		
		red	black	
Eyes	blue	10	22	32
	brown	24	9	33
		34	31	65

f. Nausea (N) & 2 drugs

		Drug A		
		No N	N	
Drug B	No N	75	13	88
	N	3	9	12
		78	22	100

g. Effect of drug on HBP

		After		
		N	Y	
Before	N	28	6	34
	Y	1	32	33
		29	38	67

7. SURVIVAL ANALYSIS

Approaches discussed in the preceding two chapters generally focused on data generated at a specific time point. An alternative design would be to observe continuously to generate data that consist of the times at which a particular class of events occurred. For example, we may be interested in comparing the times to death or relapse for patients receiving two different treatment regimens, or the latencies of a particular disease in groups of animals of various genotypes. Because the events of interest are often death or failure, this class of problems is generally referred to as *survival analysis*. However, the methods discussed in this chapter are applicable to any type of time-to-event data, such as time to flowering for two groups of plants raised under different conditions.

We could, of course, analyze our data using the categorical or rank sum methods discussed previously. For example, we could choose a fixed time point and ask whether the proportions of patients surviving to that time differed for our two treatments using Fisher's exact test or a Chi-square test. However, our result will depend on the time point we choose. Consider the case where the long-term survival of patients on the two therapies is similar, but most of the deaths of patients receiving treatment A occur soon after the start of therapy, while those on therapy B occur many months later. We would generally view the latter treatment to be superior to the former, in spite of the similar end result. Alternatively, we could treat the event times as the random variable of interest and use the Wilcoxon rank sum test to compare two groups. This approach would avoid the loss of information inherent in comparing proportions at a particular time, but still may not take full advantage of the available data. A feature of our observational design is that some patients or experimental animals may be lost before the end of the study. For example, a patient may elect to withdraw from a study or an experimental animal suffer an accidental death. Such observations are *censored* but still contain relevant information. If a subject is censored at time t, we do not know its true event time, but do know that it must be longer than t.

Because of its importance to fields ranging from industrial quality assurance to clinical research, survival analysis has been an active area of statistical research, and there are numerous books on the subject (*e.g.*, Cox and Oakes, 1984; Lee and Wang, 2003). In this chapter we will focus on just two topics, nonparametric estimation of survival distributions and tests for differences in survival between two treatment groups.

7.1. Estimating Survival Functions

Our experiment consists of n samples, each having an associated T_j, time to event, and C_j, time to censorship. The T_j and C_j are assumed to be mutually independent, *i.e.*, censoring time provides no information on the true survival time. For each sample, we observe

$$X_j = \min\{T_j, C_j\} \quad \text{and}$$

$$\delta_j = \begin{cases} 1 & \text{if } T_j \leq C_j \ (\textit{i.e.}, \text{true survival time}) \\ 0 & \text{if } T_j > C_j \ (\textit{i.e.}, \text{censored sample}) \end{cases}$$

The cumulative distribution of event times is $F(x) = P(T \leq x)$. We want to estimate the survival function, $S(x) = 1 - F(x)$.

Within our experiment, we observe k distinct failure times, which we order $t_{(1)} < t_{(2)} < \ldots < t_{(k)}$. At any given time, $t_{(i)}$, we observe d_i failures among n_i subjects at risk. A natural estimator for the probability of failing at time $t_{(i)}$ is the ratio d_i/n_i. Thus, the conditional probability of surviving past $t_{(i)}$, given that the subject has survived to that time, is $(1 - d_i/n_i)$. Multiplying the successive conditional probabilities of survival gives us the unconditional probability of survival past time $t_{(i)}$. This estimator for survival was originally described by Kaplan and Meier (1958) as the product limit estimator, and is now generally called the Kaplan-Meier estimator. Thus, the survival is estimated as

$$\hat{S}(x) = \prod_{t_{(i)} \leq x} \left(1 - \frac{d_i}{n_i}\right)$$

As above, d_i is the number of failures (events) at time i and n_i the number at risk at that time. By convention, if both failures and censored observations occur at $t_{(i)}$, the failures are assumed to occur before censoring; *i.e.*, the number of censored observations is included in n_i. Plotting $\hat{S}(x)$ as a function of time gives a stepped curve, with decreases at the distinct failure times. The curve does not change at times of censorship, but the censoring times are sometimes indicated on the survival curve by a tic mark or other symbol.

Note that the assumption specified above that censoring occurs independently of failure events is critical. If imminent failure makes it more likely that a sample will be censored, we will over-estimate survival. We can avoid this problem by properly defining the event of interest. As an obvious example, consider an experiment in which we follow the survival of animals infected with a pathogen. Deaths of individual animals would be noted as the group was inspected each morning. However, we should also humanely sacrifice those animals that are found to be moribund. These animals should not be considered censored observations; we sacrificed them because death would likely occur in a matter of hours or days. Defining our event as death or extensive morbidity would provide a better estimate of the true survival curve.

Example 7.1

You have constructed a transgenic mouse line that expresses a gene in the mammary gland that you believe will increase cancer risk. You follow a cohort of mice for up to 85 weeks, and note the time that a mammary tumor is first detected by palpation, evaluating all of the animals weekly. Among the 14 animals in the study, you observe tumors at 33, 41, 41, 55, 57, 66, 72, 73, and 84 weeks. Four animals are still tumor-free at 85 weeks and one was lost to a handling accident at 42 weeks. We can estimate the survival curve as in the table below:

Time	d_i	n_i	$(1-d_i/n_i)$	$\hat{S}(t_i)$
33	1	14	0.929	0.929
41	2	13	0.846	0.786
55	1	10	0.900	0.707
57	1	9	0.889	0.629
66	1	8	0.875	0.550
72	1	7	0.857	0.471
73	1	6	0.833	0.393
84	1	5	0.800	0.314

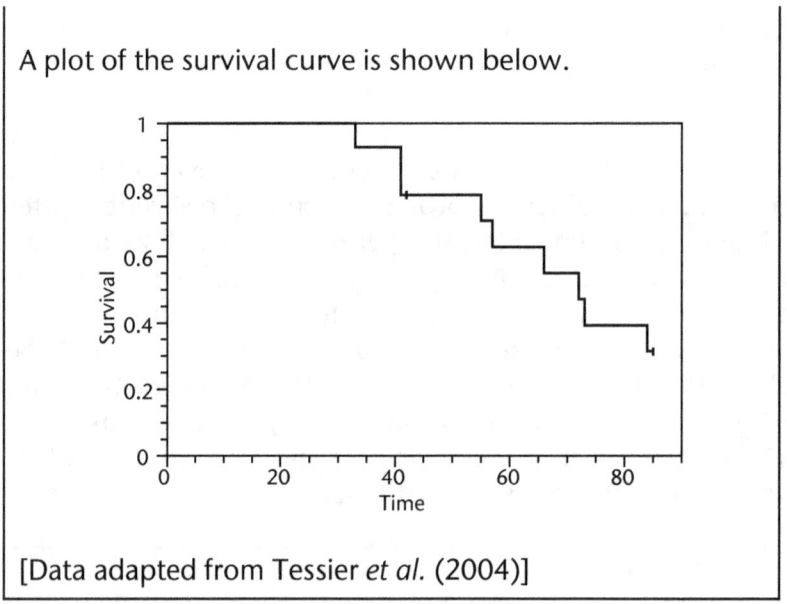

A plot of the survival curve is shown below.

[Data adapted from Tessier *et al.* (2004)]

7.1.1. Variance and confidence limits for survival.

To obtain the variance of the Kaplan-Meier estimator, we can consider the hazard function

$$\lambda(t) = \frac{f(t)}{S(t)}$$

which may be thought of as the probability that an event will occur in the interval $t + \Delta t$, given that an individual has survived to time t. The cumulative hazard function is

$$\Lambda(t) = \int_0^t \lambda(t)dt = -\ln(S(t))$$

The variance of $\Lambda(t)$ can be obtained as the sum of independent intervals:

$$V(\hat{\Lambda}(t)) = \sum_{t_i \leq t} \frac{d_i}{n_i(n_i - d_i)}$$

Given the relationship between the survival and cumulative hazard functions, we can estimate the variance of $S(t)$ as

$$V(\hat{S}(t)) = \hat{S}^2(t)V(\hat{\Lambda}(t)) \quad \text{(because V}(\ln f)=V(f)/f^2).$$

We can use a normal approximation to obtain $(1-\alpha)$ confidence limits for survival at a given time. In order to insure that our confidence limits lie between 0 and 1, we can use a *log-log* transformation of the survival curve (*i.e.*, the log hazard) and estimate the confidence limits in terms of the cumulative hazard:

$$g(t) = \ln(-\ln(\hat{S}(t))) = \ln(\hat{\Lambda}(t))$$

$$V(g(t)) = \frac{V(\hat{\Lambda}(t))}{\left(-\ln(\hat{S}(t))\right)^2}$$

Confidence limits $(1-\alpha)$ for the transformed survival are

$$g(t) \pm z_{\alpha/2} \, V(g(t))^{1/2}$$

where $z_{\alpha/2}$ is from the standard normal distribution (1.96 for the 95% confidence limits). Transforming back to the same scale as survival, we obtain confidence limits of

$$\exp(-\exp(\ln(-\ln \hat{S}(t)) \pm z_{\alpha/2} \, V(g(t))^{1/2}))$$

More complex approaches to obtaining the confidence limits for the survival curve as a whole (rather than at arbitrary time points) are also available (see Hollander and Wolfe, 1999).

Example 7.1 (continued)

Using the approximations given above, standard deviations and 95% confidence limits for the survival curve obtained in our tumor study are given by the table below.

Time	$\hat{S}(t_i)$	s.d.	95% CI
33	0.93	0.07	(0.59, 0.99)
41	0.79	0.11	(0.47, 0.92)

55	0.71	0.12	(0.39, 0.88)
57	0.63	0.13	(0.32, 0.83)
66	0.55	0.14	(0.26, 0.77)
72	0.47	0.14	(0.20, 0.70)
73	0.39	0.14	(0.15, 0.64)
84	0.31	0.13	(0.10, 0.56)

7.1.2. Median survival.

The most commonly used summary statistic for survival data is the median survival and its associated confidence limits. In the absence of censoring, or if the few censored observations occur at the end point of the experiment, we can obtain the median survival in the usual way. The n survival times are ordered (with the terminally censored observations placed at the end of the list). If the number of observations is odd, the median is $t_{(n+1)/2}$. For an even number of samples, the median is $0.5(t_{n/2}+t_{1+n/2})$.

If our experiment includes censored observations, we can estimate the median survival from the Kaplan-Meier survival curve. The median is the time of the first event at which the Kaplan-Meier estimator is below 0.5. This approach is equivalent to drawing a horizontal line at a survival of 50% on the graph of the survival curve and determining the time at which the line intersects the curve. For our Example 7.1 above, the median survival (tumor latency) is 72 weeks.

The bootstrap method provides the most robust approach to obtaining confidence limits for the median survival. Example 3.4 estimated median survival for two data sets in which no censoring had occurred. Applying the bootstrap method to randomly censored data is equally straightforward (see Efron, 1981). As discussed above, each sample in our experiment consists of two values (x_i, δ_i), where the first in the pair is the time of the event or censoring and the latter is 1 in the case of failure or 0 if the sample is censored. Each bootstrap sample is constructed by drawing n times with replacement from the set of (x_i, δ_i) pairs. The median survival is then estimated from the Kaplan-Meier estimators obtained using the bootstrap samples.

7.2. Comparing Survival Curves

Consider an experiment in which we obtain survival or event times for two groups of subjects. For example, we have developed a new therapy and want to test the hypothesis that patients receiving this treatment regimen survive longer than those treated with a standard therapy. Another example: We are studying a mutation that we suspect may delay sexual maturation in male mice. We house individual mutant or wild-type males with a pair of females and for each animal record the age of the male at the time the first litter is delivered (the event time being age at fatherhood).

The most commonly used statistical test for comparing survival curves is the logrank test, also referred to as the Mantel-Cox test (Peto and Peto, 1972). There are several different approaches to deriving this test statistic. The formulation below is simplest to compute and can easily be extended to testing the null hypothesis that three or more survival distributions are identical.

Consider two groups of observations (x_{ij}, δ_{ij}), defined as above except that the subscript i indicates the experimental group and j the sample within the group. We assume that the distributions of failure times and censoring times are mutually independent. Order the event times jointly for the two groups, yielding K distinct event times. For each of these distinct times, determine d_{ik}, the number of events in group i at time k and n_{ik}, the number of subjects at risk. For each time, k, we can construct a 2×2 table

Time k	Event	Not Event	Total
Group 1	d_{1k}	$n_{1k}-d_{1k}$	n_{1k}
Group 2	d_{2k}	$n_{2k}-d_{2k}$	n_{2k}
Total	d_k	N_k-d_k	N_k

We can compute the number of expected events at time k for each group as $E_{ik}=(n_{ik} \times d_k)/N_k$. For each group, the total number of observed events is

$$O_i = \sum_{k=1}^{K} d_{ik}$$

while the total number of expected events is

$$E_i = \sum_{k=1}^{K} \frac{n_{ik}d_k}{N_k}$$

We compute the logrank test statistic as

$$X^2 = \sum_{i=1}^{2} \frac{(O_i - E_i)^2}{E_i}$$

which follows a χ^2 distribution with 1 degree of freedom. This form of the test makes it easy to compute the hazard ratio, or relative risk, for the two treatments as

$$HR = \frac{O_1 / E_1}{O_2 / E_2}$$

This test can readily be extended to more than two groups, the number of degrees of freedom being one less than the number of groups. As formulated above, this test is two-sided; *i.e.*, the null hypothesis that the two survival distributions are identical is tested against the general alternative that they are different.

A different approach to computing the test statistic for two groups allows for a one-sided test. Compute O_1 and E_1, the observed and expected number of events for group 1, as above. The one-sided test statistic, M, which follows a standard normal distribution, is

$$M = \frac{O_1 - E_1}{\sqrt{V_1}}$$

where the variance, V_1, is

$$V_1 = \sum_{k=1}^{K} \frac{d_k(N_k - d_k)n_{1k}n_{2k}}{N_k^2(N_k - 1)}$$

Example 7.2

Extending our study of mammary tumor development in transgenic mice, we obtain a second line that expresses the transgene at higher levels than our first line. We set up cohorts of both lines and examine each animal weekly for the presence of a palpable tumor. The ages (in weeks) at tumor development in each group are given below (a '+' appended to a value indicates a censoring time):

Low expression: 30 34 40 45 56 56 56 56 63 68 78 76 80
81 82 85+ 85+ 85+ 85+ 85+ 85+ 85+ 85+
85+ 85+

High expression: 24 37 37 39 40 40 40 45 49 50 60 63 66
68 69 70 72 84 85+

The survival curves for the two groups are illustrated below:

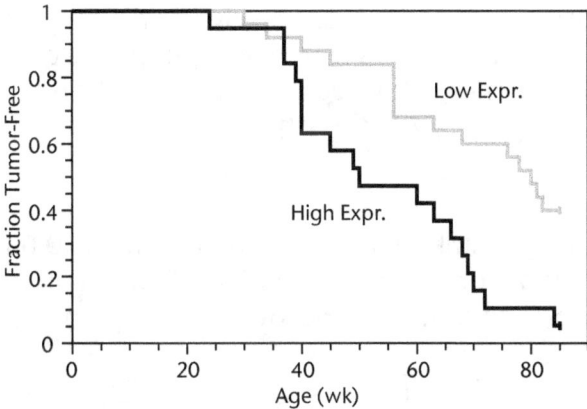

There are 23 distinct event times among the two groups. The appropriate 2×2 tables and expected number of events, E_{ik}, for the first few times are:

Time=24	Tum.	No Tum.	Total	E_{ik}
Low	0	25	25	0.568
High	1	18	19	0.432
Total	1	43	44	
Time=30	Tum.	No Tum.	Total	E_{ik}
Low	1	24	25	0.581
High	0	18	18	0.419
Total	1	42	43	

Time=34	Tum.	No Tum.	Total	E_{ik}
Low	1	23	24	0.571
High	0	18	18	0.429
Total	1	41	42	
Time=37	Tum.	No Tum.	Total	E_{ik}
Low	0	23	23	1.122
High	2	16	18	0.878
Total	2	39	41	
Time=39	Tum.	No Tum.	Total	E_{ik}
Low	0	23	23	0.590
High	1	15	16	0.410
Total	1	38	39	

The number of observed events in the low and high expression lines is 15 and 18, respectively. Summing up the expected number of events for the two groups, we get 22.978 and 10.022. Thus, the value of our test statistic is

$$X^2 = \frac{(15-22.978)^2}{22.978} + \frac{(18-10.022)^2}{10.022}$$
$$= 9.12$$

From the χ^2 distribution (1 df), we find that $P<0.003$. The hazard ratio for mammary tumor development in the high expression line relative to the low expression line is

$$HR = \frac{18/10.022}{15/22.978} = 2.8$$

[Data adapted from Tessier *et al.* (2004)]

7.3. Sample Problems

1. Plot the survival curves for the two treatment groups in Example 3.4. Is there a significant difference in survival between the two treatments?

2. You have developed a novel corn line that has been selected for earlier maturation. The new line is planted in a field together with its progenitor and the number of days to maturation is recorded for each plant. The experiment is terminated at 75 days. The results are (appended + indicates censored sample):

    | Progenitor | 55, 58, 58, 61+, 62, 62, 64, 64+, 66, 69, 70, 74, 75+, 75+ |
    | Selected Line | 48, 49, 49, 50, 52+, 58, 59, 59, 62, 64, 65, 65, 65, 66+, 68, 69, 75+ |

    Does the new line mature more rapidly than the starting line?

8. Correlation and Regression

8.1. Tests of Independence

For categorical data, Fisher's exact test (for 2×2 tables) or the Chi-Square test (for $r \times c$ contingency tables) provides a means to test for independence between the two methods of classifying a set of observations. We can generalize this problem by considering the case of making *bivariate* observations on n independent samples. That is, for each sample i ($i = 1$ ... n), we measure X_i and Y_i, where X and Y represent two different random variables. The question of interest is whether or not the X and Y random variables are associated. If the X and Y random variables could only take on values of 0 or 1, we could organize the data in the familiar 2×2 table and use Fisher's exact test for independence. We need to develop a different approach for the case that the Xs and Ys are each random variables distributed along some portion of the real line.

A familiar measure of the degree of independence of the X and Y variates is the correlation coefficient, r, which was defined by Pearson as

$$r(x,y) = \frac{E[(x-\mu_x) \times (y-\mu_y)]}{\left\{ E[(x-\mu_x)^2] \times E[(y-\mu_y)^2] \right\}^{0.5}}$$

$$= \frac{E(xy) - E(x)E(y)}{\sigma_x \sigma_y}$$

The value of r ranges from -1.0 to +1.0, depending on whether large X values are associated with small or large Y values, respectively. When X and Y are uncorrelated, the value of r is 0. This measure of correlation is sensitive to "fat tails" in the distributions of the random variables. In addition, traditional tests of the hypothesis that the value of r differs significantly from 0 are based on the assumption that both X and Y are normally distributed. In order to avoid these limitations, we can define both measures of correlation and a test of independence based on permutations of the sample ranks. It is important to point out that such a test measures only the independence of the two variates and does not address issues of causality.

8.1.1. Spearman's rank correlation coefficient.

An equivalent to Pearson's product moment correlation coefficient, r, based on sample ranks rather than the values of the observations was proposed by Spearman (1904). If $R(X_i)$ is the rank of X_i among the X values and $R(Y_i)$ the rank of Y_i among the Y values (using mid-ranks for tied values), Spearman's rank correlation coefficient is given by

$$\rho = \frac{\sum_{i=1}^{n} R(X_i)R(Y_i) - n\left(\frac{n+1}{2}\right)^2}{\left(\sum_{i=1}^{n} R(X_i)^2 - n\left(\frac{n+1}{2}\right)^2\right)^{1/2}\left(\sum_{i=1}^{n} R(Y_i)^2 - n\left(\frac{n+1}{2}\right)^2\right)^{1/2}}$$

In the case that there are no ties among the ranks, this equation simplifies to

$$\rho = 1 - \frac{6\sum_{i=1}^{n}[R(X_i) - R(Y_i)]^2}{n(n^2 - 1)}$$

The value of ρ may be used to test the hypothesis that X and Y are independent. The value

$$z = \rho\sqrt{n-1}$$

follows a standard normal distribution. Depending on the sign of ρ, the value of z will fall within the lower ($\rho < 0$) or upper ($\rho > 0$) tail of the normal distribution. For a two-sided test of independence, simply multiply the appropriate tail probability by 2. One-sided tests for positive or negative correlation are provided by the upper- and lower-tail probabilities, respectively.

Example 8.1

A series of recombinant inbred mouse strains was compared for their spontaneous incidence of liver cancer and their sen-

---

sitivities to chemically induced tumors at that site. The table below shows each phenotype (with the rank in parentheses):

Strain	Induced	Spont. (%)
3	26 (11)	27 (8)
4	6.3 (5)	82 (11)
6	1.9 (2)	4 (3.5)
7	23 (10)	26 (6.5)
8	20 (7.5)	64 (10)
9	20 (7.5)	26 (6.5)
10	4.1 (4)	7 (5)
14	2.2 (3)	3 (1.5)
19	12 (6)	3 (1.5)
C	22 (9)	52 (9)
B	1.1 (1)	4 (3.5)

Computing ρ, we obtain

$$\rho = \frac{456.75 - 396}{10.464 \times 10.416}$$
$$= 0.557$$

Thus, $z = 1.76$, and the one-sided P-value is 0.04.

[Data from Lee and Drinkwater, 1995.]

8.1.2. Kendall's test for independence.

A conceptually simpler approach, described by Kendall (1938), arises when we rephrase our hypothesis of independence as

$$H_0: P[(X_i - X_j)(Y_i - Y_j) > 0] = 0.5$$

against, for example, the two-sided alternative

$$H_2: P[(X_i - X_j)(Y_i - Y_j) > 0] \neq 0.5$$

We can use this form of the null hypothesis to define a test statistic, K, based on the $n(n-1)/2$ pairwise comparisons of the X and Y values as follows. If we define sgn(b) as the sign of b (that is, a value of -1 if the sign is negative, +1 if the sign is positive, and 0 if $b = 0$), we can compute

$$K=\sum_{i=1}^{n-1} \sum_{j=i+1}^{n} \text{sgn}[(X_i - X_j) \times (Y_i - Y_j)]$$

The value of K ranges from $-n(n-1)/2$ to $+n(n-1)/2$ for perfect negative and positive correlations, respectively. Note that by defining the test statistic in this way, we would obtain the same value whether we used the actual values of the observations or their ranks from 1 to n within the X and Y values. For small values of n we can readily compute the distribution of the test statistic under the null hypothesis of independence. If we reorder the X values by increasing rank, we can compute the value of K for all of the $n!$ permutations of the Y values by considering only the ranks of the Y variate. As an example, the permutations of the Y ranks and the distribution of K for $n = 4$ are shown below.

Permutation	K	Permutation	K
1,2,3,4	6	3,1,2,4	2
1,2,4,3	4	3,1,4,2	0
1,3,2,4	4	3,2,1,4	0
1,3,4,2	2	3,2,4,1	-2
1,4,2,3	2	3,4,1,2	-2
1,4,3,2	0	3,4,2,1	-4
2,1,3,4	4	4,1,2,3	0
2,1,4,3	2	4,1,3,2	-2
2,3,1,4	2	4,2,1,3	-2
2,3,4,1	0	4,2,3,1	-4
2,4,1,3	0	4,3,1,2	-4
2,4,3,1	-2	4,3,2,1	-6

K	p(K)
6	1/24
4	3/24
2	5/24
0	6/24
-2	5/24
-4	3/24
-6	1/24

The distribution of K for various values of n has been tabulated in Appendix 6 for a one-sided statistical test (simply double the P-values to obtain the two-sided signficance level). From above, you can see that the expected value of K is 0 and that the distribution is symmetrical. Thus, for large values of n, we can define an approximate statistic, K^*, that follows a standard normal distribution.

$$K^* = K /[n(n - 1)(2n + 5)/18]^{1/2}$$

Using the statistic K, we can define a measure, τ, of the degree of independence that is analogous to ρ defined above, such that $-1 \le \tau \le +1$,

$$\tau = 2K / n(n - 1)$$

This measure does not behave in quite the same way that r or ρ do. As a rule of thumb for evaluating (in your head only) the quality of a correlation, consider $(\tau)^{1/2}$ to be the rough equivalent to r or ρ. Hypothesis tests for independence based on K and ρ will generally give very similar results.

Example 8.2

Inbred mouse strains have characteristic patterns of tumor induction for various tissues following treatment with a chemical carcinogen. Young male animals of several inbred strains were treated with a single dose of carcinogen and the number of tumors induced in the liver and lungs of each animal was evaluated at 8 months of age. For each strain, the mean liver and lung tumor multiplicities were calculated and we want to test the hypothesis that the sensitivities for tumor induction at the two sites are independent. In the table below, the strains were ordered on the basis of the liver tumor multiplicity

Strain	Mean Tumor Multiplicity	
	Liver	Lung
SWR/J	0	16
A/J	0.2	23
C57BL/6J	0.3	1.5
C57BR/cdJ	7.1	1.0
P/J	15	1.8
SM/J	17	1.9
CBA/J	45	6.0

The ranks of the lung tumor multiplicities (ordered by increasing liver tumor multiplicity are

K	6	7	2	1	3	4	5
	-4	-5	2	3	2	1	

and the test statistic is $K = -1$ and $P = 1.0$. The value of τ is $-2/7(6) = -0.048$.

[Data adapted from Kemp and Drinkwater, 1989.]

8.2. Regression

In the discussion above, both the X and Y observations were random variables and we were interested in the degree to which the two random variables were associated or "varied together." We might also be interested in whether X and Y displayed a particular functional relationship. Estimation and hypothesis testing related to such a functional relationship can be approached by the use of regression analysis.

8.2.1. Estimation by least squares.

We will discuss only a small (but highly useful) part of the general problem of regression analysis – estimation by the method of least squares of the parameters describing a linear functional relationship between a dependent random variable Y_j and one or more independent variates X_{ij}. In the equation

$$Y_j = \beta_0 + \beta_1 x_{1j} + \beta_2 x_{2j} + \ldots + \beta_k x_{kj} + \varepsilon_j$$

Y_j represents our measured random variable (*e.g.*, weight, body length, survival), the β_i are the parameters we want to estimate, the x_{ij} are known coefficients (*e.g.*, dose of drug, age, genotype) that may be fixed by the experimental design, and ε_j is an "error" random variable. Note that by *linear* regression we are referring only to the parameters:

$$Y_j = \beta_0 + \beta_1 x_1 + \varepsilon_j$$
$$Y_j = \beta_0 + \beta_1 x_1 + \beta_2 x_1^2 + \varepsilon_j$$
$$Y_j = \beta_0 + \beta_1 \sin(x_1) + \beta_2 \cos(x_2) + \varepsilon_j$$

are all linear models while

$$Y_j = \beta_0 + \beta_1 x_1 + \beta_1^2 x_2 + \varepsilon_j$$

is not.

Estimates of the parameters, β_i, obtained by the method of least squares are unbiased, minimum variance estimators whether or not the error terms, ε_j, are normally distributed. Unfortunately, hypothesis testing (*e.g.*, that two regression lines have the same slope, that the value of the parameter β_2 is 0, *etc.*) does depend on the form of the distribution of the random variable. Thus, we will focus on the estimation problem using the method of least squares. Nonparametric methods for hypothesis testing are discussed in the next section.

The general linear regression equation above can be written in matrix notation as

$$Y = X\beta + \varepsilon$$

where Y is the ($n\times1$) vector of observations, X is an ($n\times k$) matrix of known coefficients, β is the ($k\times1$) vector of regression coefficients, and ε is an ($n\times1$) vector of "error" random variables with means and dispersion matrix E(ε)=0 and V(ε)=σ^2I (identity vector). We assume that $n\geq k$ and that $|X'X|\neq0$.

The least squares estimates of the parameters are obtained from

$$\hat{\beta} = (X'X)^{-1} X'Y$$

and an unbiased estimate of σ^2 is

$$s^2 = \frac{1}{n-k}(Y'Y - \hat{\beta}\, X'Y)$$

Using this estimate of σ^2, the variance for a particular parameter is

$$V(\hat{\beta}_i) = s^2 [(X'X)^{-1}]_{ii}$$

You can use the above results to predict the value of Y that would be obtained for a particular set of x_i conditions, represented by the vector **a**:

$$\hat{Y} = \mathbf{a}\, \hat{\beta}$$
$$V(\hat{Y}) = s^2(1 + \mathbf{a}(X'X)^{-1}\mathbf{a})$$

Example 8.3

Cultured fibroblasts are plated at low density, treated with varying doses of UV light, and allowed to grow for 2 weeks. The culture dishes are then stained and the number of colonies per dish determined. The data below are the surviving fractions (normalized to the cloning efficiency of untreated cells) as a function of dose. We want to estimate the parameters for the model

$$\log(\text{Survival}) = \beta_0 + \beta_1 \times \text{dose}$$

Dose (J/m^2)	Survival	log(Survival)
2.5	0.76, 0.85, 0.97	-0.12, -0.071, -0.013
5.0	0.67, 0.66, 0.64	-0.17, -0.18, -0.19
7.5	0.35, 0.36, 0.34	-0.46, -0.44, -0.47
10	0.19, 0.20, 0.17	-0.72, -0.70, -0.77

For a simple, straight line the parameters can be computed readily by hand using the formulas

$$\hat{\beta}_1 = \frac{n \sum x_j y_j - \sum x_j \sum y_j}{n \sum x_j^2 - \left(\sum x_j\right)^2}$$

$$\hat{\beta}_0 = \bar{y} - \hat{\beta}_1 \bar{x}$$

where the summations are over all of the observations and (in this case) y refers to the log(Survival) values and x to the UV doses.

Using the above, we find that the parameters are

$$\hat{\beta}_0 = 0.20$$
$$\hat{\beta}_1 = -0.090$$

The variances for the parameters are

$$V(\hat{\beta}_0) = \frac{s^2 \sum x_j^2}{n \sum (x_j - \overline{x})^2} = 0.0426$$

$$V(\hat{\beta}_1) = \frac{s^2}{\sum (x_j - \overline{x})^2} = 0.000908$$

where

$$s^2 = \frac{\sum (y_j - \hat{y}_j)^2}{n-2}, \hat{y}_j = \hat{\beta}_0 + \hat{\beta}_1 x_j$$

8.2.2. Nonparametric regression analysis.

For the simple linear regression problem described above, we could use Kendall's test to evaluate the correlation between UV dose and log(Survival), which would be equivalent to testing the null hypothesis that β_1 is equal to 0 against either a one- or two-sided alternative. Applying Kendall's test to the data in the example, we obtain a test statistic of $K = -54$ and a two-sided P-value of approximately 0.0002.

Theil (see Hollander and Wolfe, 1999) has extended this approach to testing the hypothesis that the slope of a straight line is equal to any specified value, m. The data consist of n observations, Y_i, each associated with an explanatory variable (which may be random or non-random), x_i. We want to test the null hypothesis that the slope β_1 is equal to a fixed value, m, against the two-sided alternative that they are not equal (or either of the one-sided alternatives). To compute Theil's statistic, first determine the differences between the observed values and that predicted by the slope under the null hypothesis

$$D_i = Y_i - mx_i \quad (i = 1 \ldots n)$$

The test statistic C is obtained from

$$C = \sum_{i=1}^{n-1} \sum_{j=i+1}^{n} \text{sgn}(D_j - D_i)$$

where, as above, sgn(a) is equal to –1 if $a<0$, 1 if $a>0$, and 0 if $a=0$. The distribution of C is identical to that for Kendall's K statistic and the same table or large sample approximation should be used. A simple distribution-free estimator for the slope can be obtained by computing the $n(n-1)/2$ individual slope estimators

$$S_{ij} = \frac{(Y_j - Y_i)}{(x_j - x_i)}, \quad 1 \le i < j \le n$$

and determining the median value. In the case that not all of the x_i are distinct, determine the median from among those values for which S_{ij} is defined. For Example 8.3, there are 54 slope estimators (excluding those with $0=x_j\text{-}x_i$) and the median value is –0.095.

8.2.3. Comparing the slopes of two or more regression lines.

As noted above, testing composite hypotheses regarding the parameters for linear regression models by the method of least squares requires that the responses are normally distributed. For the simplest regression model, that of a straight line, Sen (1969) and Adichie (1975) have proposed a nonparametric test of the hypothesis that two or more lines share a common slope, independent of the intercepts for the lines (*i.e.*, the lines are parallel).

Consider an experiment in which we want to compare the dose-responses for mutagenesis by ionizing radiation of k cell lines that are derived from patients with various alleles for loci that we suspect may influence their sensitivity to radiation-induced mutations. For each cell line, we measure the mutation frequency, Y_{ij}, at various doses, x_{ij}, of ionizing radiation ($i=1, ..., k; j=1, ..., n_i$). The responses follow the regression model

$$Y_{ij} = \beta_{0i} + \beta_{1i}x_{ij} + e_{ij}, \quad i=1...k, \quad j=1...n_i$$

We want to test the null hypothesis

$$H_0: \beta_{11} = \beta_{12} = ... = \beta_{1k}$$

against the general alternative that at least one of the slopes differs from the others.

To compute the Sen-Adichie statistic, first estimate the pooled estimator for the common slope under the null hypothesis, $\overline{\beta}$, by the method of least squares:

$$\overline{\beta} = \frac{\displaystyle\sum_{i=1}^{k}\sum_{j=1}^{n_i}(x_{ij} - \overline{x}_i)Y_{ij}}{\displaystyle\sum_{i=1}^{k}C_i^2}$$

where

$$\overline{x}_i = \sum_{j=1}^{n_i} x_{ij} / n_i$$

$$C_i^2 = \sum_{j=1}^{n_i}(x_{ij} - \overline{x}_i)^2$$

For each of the k regression lines compute the residuals

$$Y_{ij}^* = Y_{ij} - \overline{\beta}x_{ij}$$

and determine the ranks r_{ij} within the ith sample for each Y_{ij}^*. Under the null hypothesis, these ranks will be independent of x_{ij}. Next compute for each sample the sum

$$T_i^* = \sum_{j=1}^{n_i}[(x_{ij} - \overline{x}_i)r_{ij}]/(n_i + 1)$$

The Sen-Adichie statistic, V, is computed from

$$V = 12\sum_{i=1}^{k}T_i^{*2}/C_i^2$$

which follows a χ^2 distribution with k-1 degrees of freedom under the null hypothesis.

The Sen-Adichie test is appropriate only when the responses are reasonably well-modeled by a straight line, which may require transformation of the original data. In the example below, transformed data are analyzed to provide a convenient solution to the double-ratio problem, where the desired test is for the relative responses to treatment of two samples.

Example 8.4

We have observed that a novel gene we are studying is induced following treatment of cultured cells with ionizing radiation (IR) and wish to test the hypothesis that this induction is dependent on the *Atm* gene. We prepare replicate cultures for *Atm* mutant and wild type cell lines, and, for each cell line, isolate mRNA from three untreated and three irradiated cultures, and measure the level of our transcript by Northern analysis. We want to test the hypothesis that the relative responses (*i.e.*, the fold-induction) of the transcript differs for the wild type and *Atm* cell lines. Our data ($10^{-3}\times$phosphorimager counts) are

Genotype	IR	Transcript	*In* Transcript
wt	-	32,34,7	3.466,3.526,1.946
	+	128,95,111	4.852,4.555,4.710
Atm	-	48,22,41	3.871,3.091,3.714
	+	51,47,58	3.932,3.850,4.080

Using the methods described in section 3.4, we observe that IR resulted in a 4.6±2.4 fold induction in wild type cells and 1.4±0.4 fold in *Atm* cells. Do these cell lines differ in the fold-induction?

Since we have used only a single dose of ionizing radiation, we can conveniently set x_{ij} to 0 for untreated cells and 1 for treated cells. If the fold induction for the two cell lines differ, then the slopes of the log responses will differ. For both cell lines,

$$\bar{x}_i = (0+0+0+1+1+1)/6 = 0.5$$

and

$$C_i^2 = 6(\pm 0.5)^2 = 1.5$$

Using the log transcript levels and the formula given above, we obtain a common slope estimate of 1.057. The residuals for the wild type cells are (3.466, 3.526, 1.946) and (3.795, 3.497, 3.652), yielding ranks of (2, 4, 1) and (6, 3, 5), for un-treated and treated cells, respectively. Using the formula for T^*, we obtain a value of 0.5 for wild type cells. Using the same methods for *Atm* cells, the value of T^* is -0.643. Thus, the value of our test statistic, V, is 5.306. Using the χ^2 distribution with 1 df, we obtain a P-value of 0.02. Thus, we would conclude that the fold-induction for the transcript differs between the wild type and *Atm* cell lines.

8.3. Sample Problems

1. You have also measured the liver tumor multiplicities induced in female animals of the strains given in the table in Example 8.1. In the same order as the strains in the table, the mean female liver tumor multiplicities were 0, 0.05, 0.2, 5.3, 0.6, 0.1, and 0.7. Is there a significant correlation between the sexes in induced liver tumor multiplicity?

2. Epstein Barr virus (EBV) infects human B-lymphocytes and the viral genome is present as a multicopy plasmid in latently infected cells. Such cells will rarely enter the lytic cycle, producing infectious virus. The data below have been borrowed (and modified a bit) from Sugden and Metzenberg (1983), who wanted to ask whether the copy number of viral DNA and frequency of lytic growth (as measured by the production of lytic cycle antigens) were independent in a series of infected cell lines.

Cell Line	Viral DNA (copies/cell)	% Antigen positive
LCL-721	5	<0.02%
11/17-3	10	0.4
11/17-5	20	0.2
3/15-9	110	1.25
11/17-4	150	1.3
3/15-31	700	3.8

a. Are the average viral copy number and frequency of lytic growth independent?

b. Briefly state two alternative models that could account for the observed correlation.

9. Multiple Samples and Multiple Experiments

9.1. Multiple Comparisons

The methods described in the previous chapters have concentrated on comparing two independent samples for a difference in location. However, many experiments involve measurements made under a number of different conditions and we often want to make inferences regarding the relationships among these various treatment groups. Some of the relevant situations are:

1. Independent samples are obtained for a number of treatment groups and we want to test the null hypothesis that all of the treatments give the same result against an alternative that at least one pair of treatments is different in location.

2. The situation described in case (1) applies, but we wish to determine which pairs of treatments differ.

3. A number of treatments are each compared to a single control sample and we want to test, for each treatment, the null hypothesis that the treated sample is the same as the control against an alternative that they differ.

4. The treatments applied to the groups follow some natural order, *e.g.*, are part of a dose-response experiment, and we want to test the hypothesis that all of the treatments result in the same level of response against an alternative hypothesis that the response for the first treatment is less than or equal to that for the second, and the response for the second is less than or equal to that for the third, *etc.*

In case (1), the object of the experiment is to determine whether a series of treatments all give equivalent results. For example, you are concerned that some nuisance variable will affect the interpretation of subsequent experiments. For this case, the Kruskal-Wallis test (see section 5.4.1) provides an efficient approach to analyzing the data. The null hypothesis that all of the groups yield the same response may be tested against the ordered alternative described in case (4) using the Jonckheere-Terpstra test (section 5.4.2).

Cases (2) and (3) are related, differing only in the number of desired comparisons, k. For example, if we have collected data on s treatments (one of which is the control for case (3)), we want to make $k=s(s-1)/2$ comparisons for case (2), while the number of relevant comparisons is only $k=(s-1)$ for case (3). Note that the comparisons for case (3) will often be one-sided while those for case (2) would generally be two-sided. One approach to analyzing the data in these cases would be to consider each comparison independently and apply the two-sample Wilcoxon rank sum test for each relevant pair of groups. The difficulty in this approach is that we now have to consider two types of error rate for the experiment. The first, α, is the error rate per comparison, that is, the usual significance level for the two sample test. However, we also need to consider the experiment-wise error rate, α'. That these two error rates are different is obvious from considering the definition of the significance level (or P-value). Consider the case in which there are truly no differences among the treatment groups. If we set the error rate per comparison $\alpha=0.05$, the chance of falsely stating that at least one pair of groups differs increases markedly with the number of comparisons.

We are thus left with two not very satisfying alternatives. First, we could fix the value of α at some reasonable level (*e.g.*, 0.05) and run the risk of falsely stating that a particular pair of treatments differ. Alternatively, we could fix α' at some level (*e.g.*, 0.05) and avoid the above risk. However, in that case we will require so stringent an α that we would easily fail to identify two treatments that truly differ.

9.1.1. Bonferroni and related methods.

The simplest approach to taking multiple comparisons into account takes advantage of the Bonferroni inequality, which states that the experiment-wise error rate, α', is less than or equal to the sum of the k per-comparison error rates. Dividing the Type I error into equal parts, we obtain $\alpha = \alpha'/k$ as the per-comparison error rate required to achieve an experiment-wise error rate of α'. This highly conservative approach insures that the probability of incorrectly rejecting even one of the null hypotheses corresponding to our k comparisons is less than α'.

When all of the hypotheses to be tested are independent, the somewhat less conservative Dunn-Šidák method can be used (Ury, 1976). The relationship between α and α' in this case is

$$\alpha' = 1 - (1-\alpha)^k$$

or

$$\alpha = 1 - (1-\alpha')^{1/k}$$

For example, if we compare 4 treatments each to a control sample and find that one of the treatments gives a significance level smaller than our criterion of $\alpha = 0.05$, there is slightly less than one chance in five (0.19) that our assertion that the treatment is better than the control will be false. In order to obtain an experiment-wise error rate of 0.05, we would need to set the per-comparison error rate to 0.0127. Our advice (somewhat off the cuff) for dealing with this case is to perform the appropriate Wilcoxon rank sum test to compare each treatment group with the control. Any treatments with per comparison P-values less than 0.05 that would not be significant at $\alpha' = 0.1$ should be retested in a separate experiment.

In case (2) we are interested in the relationships among the various treatment groups. For this case, the number of comparisons, k, is $s(s-1)/2$. The relationship given above may be used as a guide to determining the amount of weight to be given to assertions that a particular pair of treatments differ. A reasonable way to summarize the results of multiple comparisons of this type is provided by the graphical approach shown in the example below.

Example 9.1

Consider an experiment in which plasmids expressing Neo[r] and various forms (wild type or deleted) of a transforming gene are introduced into fibroblasts. Plasmid bearing cells are selected by growth in G418 and 10^4 resistant cells are plated in agarose. The colonies in each plate are enumerated after a suitable growth period. Four plasmids are tested in multiple experiments with each assay consisting of two or more plates. The plasmids tested are SV2Neo (no transforming gene), SV2BNLF1 (wild type gene), N43b (N-terminal deletion), and C174 (C-terminal deletion). The following data are obtained.

| Expt. | No. of colonies / 10^4 cells | | | |
	SV2Neo	SV2BNLF1	N43b	C174
1	32	116	20	
	24	220	36	
	28			
	40			
2	0	405	5	35
	15	410	15	25
3	20	550	30	130
	55	735	25	160
4	70	835		820
	55	705		825
	80			
	140			
5	75	790		585
		235		340
6	40	635	125	215
	30	330	105	185
7	60	815	60	245
	90	695	75	220

[Data adapted from Baichwal and Sugden, 1989.]

The above example reflects several features of the way we actually do experiments. First, in contrast to the simple, two sample cases we have discussed so far, we were really interested in asking several different questions when we did the experiments. Second, the data were not all obtained at the same time and inspection of the data would indicate that there are systematic experiment to experiment variations. We will first deal with the multiple comparisons aspect of the first point, pooling the data across experiments. A method for analyzing the data that maintains the experiment-specific information will be discussed in section 9.2.

First consider the case of comparing three treatments against a control sample (SV2Neo). We want to test the null hypothesis that the treatment and control give the same response against an alternative that the response for the "treatment" plasmid is greater than that for SV2Neo.

Using the one-sided version of the Wilcoxon rank sum test for each of the treatments vs. control (and pooling the data across the various experiments) we obtain significance levels of $P=0.37$, $P<0.0003$, and $P<2\times10^{-6}$ for the N43b, C174, and SV2BNLF1 plasmids, respectively. At an experiment-wise error rate of $\alpha'=0.05$, we require that $\alpha<0.017$; we find that the C174 and SV2BNLF1 plasmids give greater responses than the control SV2Neo plasmid.

Next consider the more general problem of determining the relationship among the responses for all of the plasmids. Performing a two-sided Wilcoxon rank sum test for each pair of plasmids we obtain the following significance levels

	SV2Neo	N43b	C174	SV2BNLF1
SV2Neo		0.74	0.0006	3×10^{-6}
N43b			0.0014	5×10^{-5}
C174				0.048

As a convenient way to summarize the data, simply write down the group names in order of increasing response and draw a line under those pairs that fail to be significant at some level of α (*e.g.*, $\alpha=0.05$)

<u>N43b SV2Neo</u> <u>C174 SV2BNLF1</u>

For this example, the plasmids fall into three discrete groups, but note that in other cases the lines may overlap. From the discussion above, C174 would differ from the first two plasmids at an experiment-wise error rate of $\alpha'\leq0.0084$ and would differ from SV2BNLF1 with an error rate of $\alpha'\leq0.288$. Note that for an α' of 0.05, we would require $\alpha\leq0.0085$.

As noted above, the Bonferroni and Dunn-Šidák methods for controlling the experiment-wise error rate are highly conservative in that they are concerned with the general null hypothesis that all k null hypotheses corresponding to our comparisons are simultaneously true. Perneger (1998) has argued that this general null hypothesis is rarely of interest in research and points out the difficulty inherent in the decreasing power that comes from increasing the number of tests that are performed. Thus, we have the Sisyphean dilemma of greater and greater difficulty in demonstrating significant differences between groups as we study more experimental conditions. We take the middle ground in this debate. For experiments such as the one discussed in the above example, report the per comparison *P*-values. However, you should be mindful of the experiment-wise error rate. Those comparisons that would not be judged significant using an α' less than 0.1 or 0.2 (or whatever risk you're willing to take) should be re-tested in an independent study. Two alternative approaches discussed below deal with the cases that we really do care about the general null hypothesis but need improved power (*e.g.*, linkage analysis) or that we are willing to accept a certain level of false-positive results (*e.g.*, microarray analyses of gene expression).

9.1.2. Estimating experiment-wise error rates by permutation.

A more complicated problem of multiple comparisons arises in the context of linkage analysis for quantitative traits. In such experiments, we are interested in mapping the genes responsible for a quantitative trait, such as blood pressure, body weight, or the number of tumors induced in a particular tissue, to specific chromosomal regions. We perform a test cross between two inbred lines of animals (or plants), such as an N_2 backcross or F_2 intercross, and analyze all of the progeny for both the phenotype of interest and their genotypes at a large number of marker loci (often 100 or more) that are distributed across all of the chromosomes. For each marker locus, we stratify the progeny by genotype and use an appropriate statistical test to determine whether the magnitudes of the phenotype values differ among the genotypes at that marker. For example, in a backcross the test progeny will either be heterozygous or homozygous at a given marker locus for the allele carried by the recurrent parent. We could use the Wilcoxon rank sum test to compare the phenotypes of the two groups.

After performing our analyses, we have a test statistic and associated *P*-value for each marker locus. However, the hypothesis that we really want to test is whether there is a significant association between phenotype and genotype *anywhere* in the genome; *i.e.*, we want to translate our per marker *P*-values into genome-wide *P*-values. Using the approach described in the preceding sections, we could approximate the genome-wide *P*-values by multiplying the per marker *P*-values by the number of comparisons (the number of markers typed) we have performed. The problem with this approach is that our comparisons are not independent. The markers fall into linkage groups and the genotypes at linked markers are correlated. It is also important to note that the costs in time and resources of following up a spurious linkage are very high.

Churchill and Doerge (1994) provide a more satisfying, empirical approach to estimating the genome-wide P-value by permutation of the phenotype data. As above, we determine the value of our test statistic for each marker locus. We can obtain the distribution of this test statistic under the null hypothesis of no linkage between any marker and the quantitative trait locus determining our phenotype as follows. We perform a large number of Monte Carlo trials in which we randomly permute the phenotype data. For each trial, we perform the appropriate test at every marker locus and note the most extreme value obtained for the test statistic. The distribution of these extreme values approximates the distribution of our test statistic under the null hypothesis of no linkage (Lystig, 2003), providing us with an estimate of the genome-wide P-value.

Example 9.2

We have performed a backcross between two inbred mouse strains that differ in risk for liver cancer. The progeny are treated with a standard regimen to induce liver cancer, and each mouse is evaluated for the number of tumors arising in the liver and for its genotype at 103 marker loci. Data for one of the marker loci are:

Homozygotes   19 80 1 2 3 60 59 7 0 3 5 3 1
               11 23 9 25 31 58 49 12 13 6 44 18
               14 7 14 11 6

Heterozygotes 49 62 61 33 78 44 8 64 61 84 62 40
               9 21 29 14 41 35 9 32 19 38 30 19
               51 27 48 53

Using the Wilcoxon rank sum test, we obtain a normalized value for the test statistic, $W^* = -3.75$, and a per-marker P-value of 0.00018 for the two-sided test.

To obtain the genome-wide null distribution for W*, we analyze 100,000 random permutations of the tumor multiplici-
ties. The distribution of the maximum |W*| is shown in the
figure below.

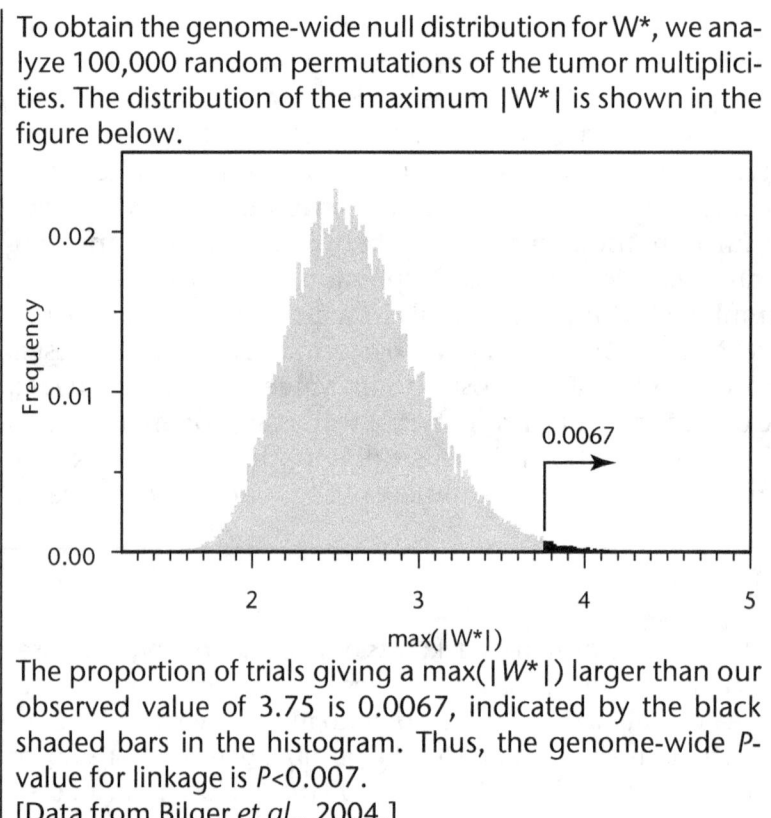

The proportion of trials giving a max($|W*|$) larger than our
observed value of 3.75 is 0.0067, indicated by the black
shaded bars in the histogram. Thus, the genome-wide *P*-
value for linkage is *P*<0.007.
[Data from Bilger *et al.*, 2004.]

9.1.3. Controlling the false discovery rate.

The application of recently developed, high throughput technolo-
gies to biological problems gives rise to issues of multiple comparisons on
an unprecedented scale. Hybridization of labeled cDNA populations, syn-
thesized from mRNA isolated from cells or tissues under various treatment
conditions, to microarrays of oligonucleotides or cDNA clones allows the
simultaneous measurement of the levels of thousands or tens of thousands of transcripts. Consider the following typical experiment to study
differential gene expression. We label mRNA samples isolated from cells
or tissues of n_1 cultures or animals treated under condition 1 and from n_2
samples under condition 2, with the conditions being, for example, two
different stages of the cell cycle, mutant and wild-type animals, *etc.* Hy-

bridization of each labeled sample to a microarray yields measurements of the levels of m transcripts. For each transcript represented on the microarray, we perform an appropriate statistical test to compare the levels under our two conditions to give m unadjusted (per comparison) P-values.

There are several noteworthy features of the above experiment. First, m is often very large. Commercially available whole genome arrays for the mouse and human allow analysis of 20,000 to 40,000 transcripts. Second, it's very likely that a large (albeit unknown) fraction of the transcripts are truly not differentially expressed. Third, the m comparisons are not independent given that many sets of genes are coordinately regulated. How do we decide which transcripts are differentially expressed?

Using the unadjusted P-values is a definite non-starter. Depending on m and the proportion of truly null comparisons, we may have up to 2,000 false positive results from our analysis among those transcripts with a per comparison P-value < 0.05. Applying the Bonferroni correction to the per comparison P-values will be far too conservative to be useful. For $m = 40,000$, we would need to set $\alpha = 1.25 \times 10^{-6}$ in order to achieve an experiment-wise error rate of $\alpha' = 0.05$. We could better estimate by permutation the distribution of our test statistic under the general null hypothesis that there are no differentially expressed genes, as in the linkage example discussed above, but that misses the point of our experiment, which is directed toward *discovering* the set of differentially regulated genes. We are likely to pursue additional studies for this set of genes, including independent measurement of the transcript levels by Northern analysis or quantitative RT-PCR, *in silico* studies of their regulatory elements, or classification of the genes into various regulatory pathways.

The methods we've discussed so far have focused on controlling the experiment-wise error rate (the probability of falsely rejecting at least one truly null hypothesis) or the per comparison error rate (the proportion of falsely rejected null hypotheses). An alternative approach to the problem of multiple comparisons has been formulated by Benjamini and Hochberg (1995). They argue that, in many circumstances, it may be more appropriate to control the false discovery rate (FDR), which is the proportion of incorrectly rejected null hypotheses among all **rejected** null hypotheses. This approach is ideal for our discovery oriented, gene expression experiment (Storey and Tibshirani, 2003). Depending on the costs associated with our follow up studies, we may be willing to tolerate a certain amount of chaff among the wheat of differentially expressed genes, to be discarded later by independent measurements of the levels of specific transcripts or representing noise in our pathway analysis.

We've performed an experiment to simultaneously test m null hypotheses, of which m_0 are true. Thus, the proportion of truly null hypotheses is $\pi_0 = m_0/m$. We can classify the results of our hypothesis tests according to the following 2×2 table:

	Declared non-significant	Declared significant	Total
True null hypotheses	$m_0 - F$	F	m_0
Non-true null hypotheses	$m - m_0 - T$	T	$m - m_0$
	$m - S$	S	m

S is an observable random variable that depends on the level α used for each individual hypothesis test. Relating these variables to the hypothesis testing framework discussed above, $E[F/m]$ is the per comparison error rate and $P(F \geq 1)$ is the experiment-wise error rate when each hypothesis is tested at a level of α'/m.

The false discovery rate, Q, is defined as

$$Q = E\left[\frac{F}{F+T}\right] = E\left[\frac{F}{S}\right]$$

with the FDR set to 0 when $S=0$, since no false rejection is possible. Benjamini and Hochberg (1995) prove two important properties of the FDR. First, when all null hypotheses are true, the FDR is equivalent to the experiment-wise error rate; thus, controlling the FDR provides a weak form of control over the experiment-wise error rate. Second, controlling the FDR at a specific level will have significantly more power than controlling the experiment-wise error rate at the same level; the power advantage to the FDR increases as m_0/m (i.e., π_0) decreases.

We want to estimate the false discovery rate, $Q(t)$, when all hypothesis tests with a P-value less than some threshold, t ($0 < t \leq 1$), are declared significant. For our m hypothesis tests, we obtain P-values of $p_1, p_2, ..., p_m$. Then

$$F(t) = \#\{\text{null } p_i \leq t; i = 1, \ldots, m\}$$
$$S(t) = \#\{p_i \leq t; i = 1, \ldots, m\}$$

When m is large,

$$Q(t) = E\left[\frac{F(t)}{S(t)}\right] \simeq \frac{E[F(t)]}{E[S(t)]}$$

The simplest estimate of $E[S(t)]$ is just the number of null hypotheses declared to be significant. The P-values for truly null hypotheses should be uniformly distributed over the interval $[0,1]$. Thus, we can estimate $E[F(t)]$ as $m_0 t = \pi_0 mt$. In the original treatment by Benjamini and Hochberg, π_0 is assumed to be 1, which yields a conservative estimate of the false discovery rate. Storey (2002) provides two alternative methods to estimate π_0 from the distribution of the P-values, but we'll use the simpler, conservative approach below.

Using the above, we can define a Q-value, q_i, for each of the P-values obtained in our experiment in a straightforward way. Order the P-values from smallest to largest, such that

$$p_1 \leq p_2 \leq \cdots \leq p_i < p_{i+1} \leq \cdots \leq p_m$$

(note the strict less than relationship above; the same Q-value will apply to all of the members of a set of equal P-values, with i taken as the largest of the set). The Q-values are estimated as

$$q_i = \frac{m \cdot p_i}{i}$$

The Q-value, q_i, is an upper limit for the false discovery rate when the P-value, p_i (and all of the tests with smaller P-values), is declared to be significant and provides a measure of the confidence we can have in asserting that gene i is, in our example, differentially expressed.

Example 9.3

We want to determine the influence of growth hormone signaling on hepatic gene expression. Hepatic mRNA was isolated from 3 wild type and 5 (growth hormone deficient) mutant mice and labeled cDNA was hybridized to a microar-ray containing sequences representing 4,608 genes. For each gene, the null hypothesis of equivalent expression in mutant and wild-type was tested using a linear model to give a moderated t-statistic (Smyth, 2004). The resulting P-values were ordered from smallest to largest. For our exper-iment, 835 genes gave per comparison P-values less than 0.05. A subset of the results are shown in the table below, with i representing the rank of the gene; p_i the unadjusted, per-comparison P-value; q_i the false discovery rate; and BP the Bonferroni adjusted P-value.

i	Clone	p_i	q_i	BP
1	4589	9.9×10^{-56}	4.6×10^{-52}	4.6×10^{-52}
2	2079	1.3×10^{-52}	3.0×10^{-49}	5.9×10^{-49}
3	540	2.5×10^{-50}	3.9×10^{-47}	1.2×10^{-46}
$\vdots$				
265	4598	9.8×10^{-6}	1.7×10^{-4}	0.045
266	3703	1.0×10^{-5}	1.8×10^{-4}	0.047
267	1294	1.2×10^{-5}	2.0×10^{-4}	0.053
$\vdots$				
561	19	5.9×10^{-3}	0.048	1
562	1266	6.0×10^{-3}	0.050	1
563	3719	6.2×10^{-3}	0.051	1

Clone 3703, which gave the 266th smallest P-value of 1.03×10^{-5}, is the last gene that would be judged significant using the Bonferroni adjusted P-values ($p_i \times 4608$). The false discovery rate for this clone is

$$q_i = \frac{4608 \times 1.03 \times 10^{-5}}{266}$$
$$= 1.78 \times 10^{-4}$$

Use of the Bonferroni adjustment would dictate that only 266 genes showed significant differential expression. Using a false discovery rate of 0.05, we would be interested in 562 genes. Our follow-up studies would likely find that approximately 28 of these 562 were not expressed at different levels in wild-type and mutant livers.

9.2. Combining Results of the Same Type

We quite frequently perform multiple independent experiments for both practical reasons and to insure that the result of an experiment is reproducible. It would be desirable to be able to jointly analyze the results of, for example, multiple experiments comparing two treatment conditions to give a single *P*-value that reflects the significance of the results as a whole. The following sections describe approaches to combining the results of replicate experiments involving measurement or categorical data.

9.2.1. Combining rank sum tests.

Consider a simple case in which we have performed s experiments and we have n_i observations for treatment 1 and m_i observations for treatment 2 ($i=1 \ldots s$), giving a total of N_i observations in experiment i. Within each experiment, the number of possible permutations of the data is $N_i!/[n_i!(N_i-n_i)!]$ and the total number of permutations for the set of experiments would be the product of this value over the s experiments. We could construct a test based on enumerating this set of permutations (at a cost of some effort), but a simpler approach, suggested by Lehman (1998), is to take advantage of the normal approximation to the Wilcoxon rank sum statistic and the properties of the normal distribution.

As above, we have performed s experiments comparing two treatments, with n_i observations on treatment 1 for experiment i and a total of $n_i+m_i=N_i$ observations in that experiment. For each experiment i, compute the Wilcoxon rank sum statistic W_i in the usual way and calculate an adjusted statistic

$$W^{(i)} = W_i / (N_i+1)$$

[The weighting by $(N_i+1)^{-1}$ provides a more powerful test for the case that the sizes of the individual experiments differ.]

The expected value and variance of $W^{(i)}$ are

$$E(W^{(i)}) = E(W_i)/(N_i+1)$$
$$V(W^{(i)}) = V(W_i)/(N_i+1)^2$$

where the expected value and variance of W_i are as given previously (see section 5.2.2). For the set of experiments as a whole, we define the statistic

$$W = \sum_{i=1}^{s} W^{(i)}$$

Because each of the $W^{(i)}$ are normally distributed, the statistic W is normally distributed with

$$E(W) = \sum_{i=1}^{s} E(W^{(i)})$$

and

$$V(W) = \sum_{i=1}^{s} V(W^{(i)})$$

Thus, the usual z-statistic $(W-E(W)]/V(W)^{0.5})$ can be used to determine the significance level.

Example 9.4
Consider the data for the two plasmids C174 and SV2BNLF1 from the example given above. These two plasmids were compared in 6 independent experiments (Experiments 2-7)

Experiment	C174	SV2BNLF1
2	25,35	405,410
3	130,160	550,735
4	820,825	835,705
5	340,585	235,790
6	185,215	330,635
7	220,245	695,815

For each of the experiments, n_i is 2 and N_i is 4. We can compute the appropriate rank sums for the experiments as follows.

Experiment	W_i	$W^{(i)}$
2	3	0.6
3	3	0.6
4	5	1.0
5	5	1.0
6	3	0.6
7	3	0.6

Thus, for this set of experiments, the value of the statistic W is 4.4. Because each experiment is of the same size, the values of $E(W^{(i)})$ and $V(W^{(i)})$ are in each case 1 and 0.0667, respectively, giving $E(W)=6$ and $V(W)=0.4$. The value of the normalized statistic is

$$z = (4.4-6) / 0.4^{1/2} = -2.52$$

and the significance level for the two-sided test is $P<0.012$. Note that by preserving the distinctions between experiments, we obtain an α that is more significant than that required for $\alpha'<0.072$, giving us some confidence that these mutant and wild-type plasmids differ in activity.

9.2.2. Combining replicate 2 × 2 tables.

Combining the results of replicate $r \times c$ tables for a general test of independence is straightforward, given the reproductive property of the χ^2 distribution. For k replicate tables, each with d degrees of freedom, the overall result can be obtained by simply summing the values of the X^2 statistics for the tables. This sum also follows a χ^2 distribution, with kd degrees of freedom.

This approach is less satisfactory when testing the hypothesis that success probabilities differ for two treatments and the goal is to combine the results of replicate 2 × 2 tables. Consider a set of k experiments in which we are comparing the success probabilities for two treatments, A and B. For each experiment, i, we obtain a table (note the difference in notation from that in Chapter 6):

Treatment	Success	Failure	Total
A	x_i	$r_i - x_i$	r_i
B	$c_i - x_i$	$N_i - r_i - c_i + x_i$	$N_i - r_i$
Total	c_i	$N_i - c_i$	N_i

We want to test the null hypothesis

$$H_0: p_{Ai} = p_{Bi} \text{ for all } i = 1 \ldots k$$

against the one-sided alternative that $p_{Ai} > p_{Bi}$ for at least some i, or the two-sided alternative that they are unequal for some i.

Mantel and Haenszel (1959) have derived the following test statistic

$$M = \frac{\sum_{i=1}^{k} x_i - \sum_{i=1}^{k} \frac{r_i c_i}{N_i}}{\left(\sum_{i=1}^{k} \frac{r_i c_i (N_i - r_i)(N_i - c_i)}{N_i^3} \right)^{0.5}}$$

The test statistic, M, follows a standard normal distribution.

Example 9.5

Mice heterozygous for a mutant allele of a particular signal transduction gene occasionally exhibit a neurological defect—their whiskers twitch more rapidly than wild type mice. The mutant mouse line is carried by three separate laboratories. Each group observes a sample of heterozygous mutant and wild type mice and a member of the group (who doesn't know the genotype) scores each mouse as a "twitcher" or normal. The null hypothesis is that the frequency of twitchers is the same for both genotypes, and the one-sided alternative is that they are more frequent among the mutants.

Results for the three groups are

Lab. A

Genotype	*Twitcher*	*Normal*	*Total*
Mutant	1	24	25
Wild type	0	20	20
Total	1	44	45

Lab. B

Genotype	*Twitcher*	*Normal*	*Total*
Mutant	4	28	32
Wild type	0	50	50
Total	4	78	82

Lab. C

Genotype	*Twitcher*	*Normal*	*Total*
Mutant	6	34	40
Wild type	1	37	38
Total	7	71	78

Using the Mantel-Haenszel test, our test statistic is

$$M = \frac{11-\left(\dfrac{25\times1}{45}+\dfrac{32\times4}{82}+\dfrac{40\times7}{78}\right)}{\left[\dfrac{25\times1\times20\times44}{45^3}+\dfrac{32\times4\times50\times78}{82^3}+\dfrac{40\times7\times38\times71}{78^3}\right]^{0.5}}$$

$$= 3.20$$

Using the table for the standard normal distribution, the *P*-value is 0.00069.

9.3. Combining Results of "Different" Types

The previous section described an approach to combining the results of several experiments in which the same statistical hypothesis was tested using the Wilcoxon rank sum test. However, there will often be a variety of experimental (and, hence, statistical) approaches to asking the same, underlying biological questions and it is desirable on scientific grounds to pursue multiple independent ways of testing our biological hypothesis. Methods for combining and interpreting the results of multiple experiments with diverse designs fall under the heading of "meta-analysis." Although meta-analysis has been an area of intense interest in recent years, in particular in its application to clinical trials, part of its origins can be traced to a very simple method proposed by R. A. Fisher in his classic "Statistical Methods for Research Workers," which was first published in 1925 (Fisher, 1973).

We have performed a number, s, of independent experiments that share the same "biological" null hypothesis and have, in each case, performed an appropriate statistical test providing us with a P-value, p_i, i.e., the probability of obtaining our observed (or a more extreme) outcome under the condition that the null hypothesis is true. As described by Fisher, we can define a test statistic that allows us to combine these independent probabilities to yield an overall test for significance:

$$X^2 = -2 \times \sum_{i=1}^{s} \ln p_i$$

This test statistic follows a χ^2-distribution with $2s$ degrees of freedom.

Example 9.6

We want to test the hypothesis that a particular mutant gene *tu* increases the risk that mice will develop lung cancer when exposed to a specific carcinogenic treatment. In order to test that hypothesis, we perform two experiments in which we treat backcross or intercross animals, genotype them at the *tu* locus, and enumerate lung tumors.

The lung tumor multiplicities for the backcross were:

tu / +   28 42 75 0 36 0 2 44 69 57 30 39 7 5 25
           2 8 50 3 10 44 0 12 29

+ /+   23 8 8 7 5 16 8 16 5 45 47 45 5 13 3 4 4
           3 4 5 15 3 2 25 26 25 5 0 11 0 47 29

Using the Wilcoxon rank sum test, we obtain a value for the normalized test statistic of $z = 1.385$, and a P-value for our one-sided test of 0.083.

The lung tumor multiplicities for the intercross were:

+ / +   76 8 25 53 108 81 26 1 139 1 13 10
         17 1 21 103 3 51 11 14 4 46

tu / +   22 47 24 5 72 11 93 57 84 18 37 47 62 12
          6 53 86 1 30 4 27 14 28 62 0 4 19 54 22 6 67

tu / *tu* 59 37 57 72 93 27 4 68 20 96 98 56 63

Using the Jonckheere-Terpstra test against the alternative that the tumor yield increases with the number of *tu* alleles, we obtain a z of 2.159 and a P-value of 0.0154.

To combine the results of these experiments we use

$$X^2 = -2 \ (\ln 0.083 + \ln 0.0154)$$
$$= -2 \ (-2.489 \ -4.173)$$
$$= 13.32$$

Using the table of the χ^2 distribution with 4 degrees of freedom, we obtain a combined P-value of 0.0098.

The above method for jointly analyzing experiments is quite powerful and can even be applied when the type of data collected in individual experiments is very different. In our example above, we could have used a different treatment protocol for the intercross that yielded a mean tumor multiplicity that was much less than 1. Thus, the data collected in that cross could have been tumor incidence as a function of genotype rather than tumor multiplicity and we may have analyzed those data using a contingency table. You would, of course, need to apply some judgment in using this approach. It seems unreasonable to combine the P-values in this way when they are derived from a two-sided statistical test and the direction of the results differs among the experiments (for example, if the backcross demonstrated a decrease in tumor yield in the presence of the *tu* allele but the intercross showed increasing yield with an increased number of copies of that allele).

9.4. Sample Problems

1. You are interested in a gene that you believe may be expressed in a
    temporally specific manner during development. In a fairly crude
    initial experiment, you isolate mRNA from embryos of various stages
    and measure the amount of transcript for the gene by Northern
    hybridization. You obtain the data below, which are obtained by
    densitometry of an autoradiogram.

    Analyze these data as completely as you can. State the hypotheses you
    are testing and compute the significance levels.

Experiment	Day of Gestation	RNA Level
1	12	20,35,33
	14	50,48,30
	16	60,31,90
	18	12,22,18
2	12	3,2,0
	14	8,7,10
	16	19,12,9
	18	0,1,2
3	12	40,45,49
	14	130,150,144
	16	220,120,350
	18	25,33,41

2. You are studying the effect of folate deficiency on the incidence of
    neural tube defects in a particular mutant mouse. You provide moth-
    ers with a folate-deficient or normal diet and analyze the embryos for
    neural tube defects. For two independent experiments, your results
    are:

Diet	NT defect	Normal
Experiment 1		
Control	0	22
Folate Deficient	3	15
Experiment 2		
Control	1	42
Folate Deficient	7	55

Does folate deficiency increase the incidence of neural tube defects in these mice?

10. POWER AND EXPERIMENTAL DESIGN

We have generally considered statistical approaches to testing hypotheses underlying a particular experiment in a *post hoc* manner. However, this way of looking at statistics does not reflect the reality of doing (or trying to do) good science. Prior to performing an experiment directed toward determining the difference between two treatments you should ask yourself two questions. First, what is the smallest level of difference between the two treatments that I would find biologically interesting? The answer to this question depends on the kind of measurement you are making, the biology of the system you are studying, and a fair bit on your emotional outlook. Second, how large an experiment must I perform in order to have a reasonable chance of reliably detecting the above difference? This second question is the key issue in experimental design and the answer depends on the statistical method to be used and on the structure of the data obtained in the experiment. We will consider these issues for three commonly used tests, Fisher's exact test for categorical data, McNemar's test for association, and the Wilcoxon rank sum test.

As discussed earlier in the course, there are two errors associated with hypothesis testing. The Type I error, α, is the probability of incorrectly **rejecting** the null hypothesis and is the commonly quoted P-value or significance level for the test. The distributions under the null hypothesis of the test statistics we have discussed are generally quite simple and do not depend on the underlying distributions of the data obtained in an experiment. The Type II error, β, is the probability of incorrectly **accepting** the null hypothesis. In order to evaluate β, or the power $(1-\beta)$, for a particular experiment we need additional information regarding the alternative hypothesis. The distribution of the test statistic under the alternative hypothesis depends on the desired value of α, the sample sizes, the distributions of the measurements, and the degree of difference between the two groups. The distribution of a test statistic under the alternative hypothesis is often referred to as its non-central distribution.

10.1. Fisher's Exact Test

Consider an experiment in which we have obtained 20 observations each on two treatments A and B and we classify each observation as a success or failure according to some criterion. We are interested in testing the null hypothesis that p_1, the probability of success for treatment A, is the same as p_2, the probability of success for treatment B, against a one-sided alternative hypothesis that $p_1 > p_2$. We have obtained the following data.

Treatment	Result		Total
	Success	Failure	
A	10	10	20
B	4	16	20
Total	14	26	40

Keeping the marginal totals fixed, the distribution of the number of successes in treatment A (x) under the null hypothesis follows a hypergeometric distribution. Using Fisher's exact test, we sum up the probabilities for x=10, 11, 12, 13, and 14 to obtain a significance level of 0.048.

The statistical model for this experiment is that the data for each treatment follow binomial distributions with success probabilities p_1 and p_2 and numbers of trials N_1 and N_2, respectively. The distribution of the test statistic under the alternative hypothesis depends on these 4 parameters and is quite difficult to evaluate. One point of relationship between α and β is that, under conditions that the statistical test gives rise to a significance level of exactly α, the power of the experiment is equal to 0.5. Casagrande *et al.* (1978) have provided an approximate formula for determining the number of observations required ($N=N_1=N_2$) to obtain a significance level α for a given β as a function of p_2 and p_1-p_2. In the table below, we have computed the equal sample sizes required for α=0.05 and β=0.1 (90% power) as a function of p_1 for various values of p_2. From the table, we can note that approximately 70 observations per group are required to obtain a 90% chance of observing a significance level ≤ 0.05 when, as in the above example, p_2=0.25 and p_1=0.5. Suissa and Shuster (1985) provide a table of sample sizes required to achieve 80% power when Barnard's exact test is used. Generally 10-20% fewer samples are required for Barnard's test relative to Fisher's exact test.

Sample sizes (per group) required for $\alpha = 0.05$, $\beta = 0.1$ for Fisher's Exact Test.
The upper and lower entries are for one- and two-sided tests, respectively.

	$p_1=0.1$	0.2	0.3	0.4	0.5	0.6	0.7	0.8	0.9	1.0
p_2										
0.05	513	94	45	28	19	14	11	8	6	5
	620	113	54	33	23	17	13	10	7	5
0.1		236	76	40	25	18	13	9	7	5
		286	92	48	30	21	15	11	9	6
0.25			1404	178	70	38	23	16	11	8
			1713	216	85	45	28	19	13	9
0.5						442	111	48	26	15
						537	134	58	31	18
0.75								1232	121	36
								1503	146	43

10.2. McNemar's Test

Consider the case-control experimental design discussed in section 6.3.1, often used to assess the association between genotype, environmental exposures, or other potential risk factors and the development of a specific disease. In our earlier example, we were interested in testing for an association between a particular genotype, G, and disease. The resulting 2×2 table, in terms of cell probabilities is:

Cases

		G	Not G	Total
	G	p_{11}	p_{01}	$p_0=p_{11}+p_{01}$
Controls	Not G	p_{10}	p_{00}	$q_0=1-p_0$
	Total	$p_1=p_{11}+p_{10}$	$q_1=1-p_1$	1

To design our study, we need to know how many cases to include in order to achieve a specific power, 1-β, for a given α, prevalence of the genotype in the controls, p_0, and odds ratio, ψ.

For this discussion, we make two simplifying assumptions. First, we will match a single control to each case. Second, the genotypes of the cases and controls are uncorrelated. Under the latter assumption of independence, the cell probabilities are determined by the marginal probabilities, *i.e.*, $p_{11}=p_1 p_0$.

We can specify all of the probabilities in the table in terms of the prevalence of the genotype in the controls, p_0, and odds ratio, $\psi=p_{10}/p_{01}$. Thus, p_1 is given by

$$p_1 = \frac{\psi p_0}{\psi p_0 + q_0}$$

For a two-sided test, the number of discordant pairs required to detect an odds ratio, ψ, with power, 1-β is (Dupont, 1988)

$$m = \frac{\left[0.5\, z_{\alpha/2} + z_\beta \sqrt{\psi/(1+\psi)^2} \right]^2}{\left[\dfrac{\psi}{1+\psi} - \dfrac{1}{2} \right]^2}$$

The number of cases required is

$$N = \frac{m}{p_{01}+p_{10}} = \frac{m}{p_0(1-p_1)+p_1 q_0}$$

(use the expression for p_1 given above to obtain N in terms of p_0 and ψ).

Example 10.1

The genotype of interest is present at a frequency of 20% in the population. How many cases are required to detect an odds ratio of 4 with 90% power (α=0.05)?

For this example, $z_{\alpha/2}$=1.96 and z_β=1.28. The number of discordant pairs required is

$$m = \frac{\left[\frac{1.96}{2} + 1.28\sqrt{\frac{4}{5^2}}\right]^2}{\left[\frac{4}{5} - \frac{1}{2}\right]^2}$$

$$= 24.7$$

The value of p_1 is

$$p_1 = \frac{4 \times 0.2}{(4 \times 0.2) + 0.8} = 0.5$$

Thus, the number of cases required is

$$N = \frac{24.7}{(0.2 \times 0.5) + (0.5 \times 0.8)}$$

$$= 49.4$$

and we should design our study to include 50 cases.

10.3. Wilcoxon Rank Sum Test

Consider two samples, each of size N, with $f_1(x)$ the distribution of the data for group 1 and $f_2(y)$ that for group 2. In the Mann-Whitney form of the test we want to evaluate the null hypothesis

$$H_0: \ P(X_i > Y_j) = 0.5$$

against the one-sided alternative

$$H_1: \ P(X_i > Y_j) > 0.5$$

The test statistic in this case is

$$W_{XY} = \text{number of pairs for which } (X_i > Y_j)$$

We can use a normal approximation to the test statistic

$$W_{XY}^* = W_{XY} - E(W_{XY}) / V(W_{XY})^{1/2}$$

In the absence of tied observations (continuously distributed data)

$$E(W_{XY}) = N^2 / 2$$

and

$$V(W_{XY}) = N^2(2N+1) / 12$$

Under the alternative hypothesis, the normalized test statistic follows a non-central t-distribution. The critical values, z', from this distribution for one-sided and two-sided tests with $\alpha=0.05$ are

Power	0.5	0.8	0.9	0.95
one-sided	1.645	2.486	2.926	3.290
two-sided	1.96	2.8	3.24	3.6

Using a little algebra, we can approximate N as a function of $P(X_i > Y_j)$ (which we will symbolize as P) for any value of z' given $\alpha=0.05$. Noting that

$$W_{XY} = N^2 P$$

we obtain

$$N \approx \{2\, z'^2\} / \{12(P-0.5)^2\}$$

For discretely distributed data in which tied observations will be frequent (*e.g.*, Poisson distributions with relatively small means), remember to add 1/2 the frequency of ties to the quantity $P(X_i > Y_j)$. In addition, the quantity "2" in the numerator of the above expression should be adjusted downward by a small amount (usually 10% or less) to take into account the reduction in variance.

Example 10.2

You want to compare two Poisson populations under conditions where you will achieve 95% power (one-sided $\alpha=0.05$) for a mean in the first sample of 2.0 against a second sample with a mean of 1.0. The distributions of the observations for the two samples is

	Frequency	
i	$m=2.0$	$m=1.0$
0	0.135	0.368
1	0.271	0.368
2	0.271	0.184
3	0.180	0.061
4	0.090	0.015
5	0.036	0.003
6	0.012	0.0005
7	0.003	7×10^{-5}

To compute

$$P(X_i > Y_j) = \left\{ \sum_{i=1}^{\infty} \left[f_1(i) \times \sum_{j=0}^{i-1} f_2(j) \right] \right\} + 0.5 \times \sum_{t=0}^{\infty} \left(f_1(t) \cdot f_2(t) \right)$$

For the two distributions above, the value of P is 0.710. Thus,

$$N = 2 \times 3.29^2 / 12 \times 0.210^2 = 41$$

If a full correction for ties is applied (and more values of i used), the value would be 38.

Example 10.3

How many observations would be required to distinguish in a two-sided test between two Poisson populations with means of 10 and 5, respectively, under conditions of 90% power with $\alpha=0.05$?

The distribution of the X_i in this case is approximately normal with mean and variance of 10, while that for the Y_j is normal with mean and variance of 5. In order to compute P, we can note that the distribution of $X-Y$ is approximately normal with a mean of 5 and a variance of 15. Using the standard cumulative normal distribution for $z=5/15^{1/2}$, we note that

$$P[(X-Y)>0] = P(X_i>Y_j) = N(1.29) = 0.901$$

Thus,

$$N = 2 \times 3.24^2 / 12 \times 0.401^2 = 11$$

10.4. Sample Problems

1. You will be comparing the cloning efficiency (colony forming ability) of two cell lines in agarose. To do this experiment, you plate 100 cells in each of N wells for each cell strain and for each well count the number of colonies that arise after 2 weeks in culture. You will compare the cloning efficiencies of the two cell strains by testing for a difference in the colony counts using the Wilcoxon rank sum test. If past experience indicates that the cloning efficiency of Cell Strain A is 10%, how many wells would you have to plate (how large must N be) in order to detect a significant difference between the two strains at the 5% significance level with power of 95% if the true cloning efficiency of Cell Strain B were 20%?

2. You are interested in studying the effect of treatment of a cell line with a hormone on the expression of an enzyme activity. The basal level of expression for the cell line is 100 units. How many independent observations (equal numbers for control and hormone-treated) would you need to make in order to have a 95% chance of detecting a two-fold increase in enzyme activity in the hormone treated cells? Assume that your measurements are normally distributed with a variance in each case of 1/2 the mean number of units.

3. The incidence of lung tumors in untreated mice of a particular strain is 10%. How many animals would you need to study in order to detect with 90% power (for $\alpha = 0.05$) an increase in tumor incidence to 30% for animals treated with a carcinogen (assume that the treated and concurrent control groups are of equal size).

APPENDICES

Appendix 1. Answers to Selected Problems

Chapter 1.

1. Their conclusions are identical.
2. No, these are opposite conclusions.
3. (Note: ~ is 'not' and ? is 'maybe'): ~M,~F; ~M,?F; ?M,~F; ?M,?F; ~(MF).
4. Answer: 3^5
5. Answer: 1/3
6. Answer: 6.
7. Answer: 60.
8. Answer: 3/4.
9. a. P(AB)=0.15, P(A)=0.50, P(B)=0.30, P(AB)=P(A)P(B), yes.; b. P(Bc)=0.15, P(B)=0.30, P(c)=0.70, P(Bc)≠P(B)P(c), no.; c. P(A|B) = P(AB)/P(B)=0.15/0.30=1/2.; d. 1/3; e. 0.2857; f. no.
10. Answer: P = 1.0.
11. Answers: *b.* p^4 *c.* p^2q^2 *d.* 1/4 *e.* p *f.* p^2 *g.* $3p^2q^2/(1-q^2)$ *h.* p^2 *i.* $1-p^2$
12. Answer: $\binom{n}{2} 3^{n-2}$
13. Answers: 20! / (5! 6! 4! 3!); 18! / (4! 5! 4! 3!)

Chapter 2.

1. Mean, 3.704; Variance, 4.427
3. The required probability is P(no females) + P(all females), or $P=2 \times 0.5^6 = 0.03125$.
4. For a Poisson distribution with mean 15, the probability of getting 25 or more mutants is $p = 1 - P(x \le 24 | m = 15) = 0.0112$.
5. a) Given that $p=0.5$, we want a value of N that will insure that P(s=0)≤ 0.05. For N = 4, P(0)=0.0625 and N=5, P(0)=0.03125; we should use 5 animals. b) After 5 generations, the chance that it won't be lost is $(1-0.03125)^5 = 0.853$.
6. The chance that an individual cell will carry B is 0.092. If the two markers were independent, the probability (from the binomial distribution) of 8 or more B+ cells with N=10 and p=0.092 is about 2×10^{-7}.
7. Under the null hypothesis, the probability that, in a given pair, the X carrier would show a higher value is 0.5. For the 8 lines tested, 6 gave a

higher value in the presence of X. From the binomal distribution $P(s \geq 6|N=8, p=0.5)=0.145$.

8. For $m=1$ and $x \geq 2,3,$ and 4, the exact probabilities are 0.264, 0.080, and 0.019 while the normal approximation (with continuity correction) gives 0.309, 0.067, and 0.0062. For $m=8$ and $x \geq 11,14$, and 16, exact probabilities are 0.184, 0.034, and 0.008 while approximate probabilities are 0.188, 0.026 and 0.004.

9. The distribution will be the sum of the three Poisson distributions, with the heterozygote accounting for 1/2 the density.

Chapter 3.

2. First find the MLE of $\Theta = (1 - r)^2$. You should get 0.4835. From this you can find the estimate of r to be 0.3047. Then calculate its variance which is given by $V(\Theta) = \dfrac{2\Theta(1-\Theta)(2+\Theta)}{n(1+2\Theta)} = 0.002174$. Then from the large sample variance formula for a transformed variable, $\dfrac{1}{V_r} = \dfrac{1}{V_\Theta}\left(\dfrac{d\Theta}{dr}\right)^2$, derive the variance of $\hat{r}$ to be 0.001124.

3. The mean number of clones per filter is 19.8. Using the bootstrap method, we obtain 95% confidence limits of (17.4, 22.2).

4. The mean (sd) for the three mutants are 0.458 (0.104), 1.82 (0.490), 0.149 (0.119), respectively.

5. The mean (variance) by the exact and approximate methods are 4.22×10^6 (4.80×10^{13}) and 1.80×10^6 (1.08×10^{13}), respectively.

Chapter 4.

1. The power is 0.98.

2. Testing on D/D, P=0.091; testing on d/d, P=0.041. For the D/D, the critical values and power are as in the example. For the d/d test, the critical value is 9 and the power is 0.69.

Chapter 5.

1. Using the Wilcoxon signed rank test, $W_s = 8$ for the negative values and $P=0.348$.

2. For the one-sided test, W=28 and P=0.0318.

3. Using the Kruskal-Wallis test, $X^2 = 17.42$, P=0.0006

4. Using the one-sided Wilcoxon rank sum test, $P < 6 \times 10^{-3}$.
5. Using the Jonckheere-Terpstra test, $z=4.20$ and the one-sided P-value is 1.3×10^{-5}.

Chapter 6.
1. Using a two-sided Fisher's exact test, $P=0.193$.
2. $X^2=2.63$, $P=0.104$
3. $X^2=2.84$, 2 degrees of freedom; $P=0.242$.
4. $X^2=12.37$, 6 degrees of freedom; $P=0.055$.
5. This is an example of Simpson's paradox. The dependence of the frequency of death penalty verdicts reverse when the combined table is compared with the tables stratified by victim race.
6. *a*. Fisher's exact test, $P=0.33$; *b*. Fisher's exact, $P=0.81$; *c*. $X^2=19.86$, 1 df, $P<10^{-5}$; *d*. Fisher's exact, $P=0.01$; *e*. $X^2=11.2$, 1 df, $P=0.0008$; *f*. McNemar's test, $P=0.02$; *g*. McNemar's test, $P=0.125$.

Chapter 7.
1. $X^2 = 9.71$, $P = 0.0018$.
2. $X^2 = 1.67$, $P = 0.20$

Chapter 8.
1. $K=11$, $n=7$, $P=0.068$.
2. $K=11$, $n=6$, $P=0.0146$.

Chapter 9.
1. Using the Kruskal-Wallis test, we obtain X^2 values of 6.90, 9.12, and 9.05 for the three experiments (each with 3 df); P-values are 0.075, 0.028, and 0.029. Combining these experiments, we get $X^2=25.06$ (9 df) and $P=0.0029$.
2. Using the Mantel-Haenszel test, we get a test statistic of –2.49 and a two-sided P-value of 0.013.

Chapter 10.
1. Using the normal approximation $P(X>Y)=0.966$; approximately 10 wells per group would be required for the two-tailed test.
2. 8 observations per group.
3. From the table, 76 per group for the one-sided test.

Appendix 2. Cumulative Normal Distribution (upper tail)

x	0	0.01	0.02	0.03	0.04	0.05	0.06	0.07	0.08	0.09
0	0.5	0.496011	0.492022	0.488033	0.484047	0.480061	0.476078	0.472097	0.468119	0.464144
0.1	0.460172	0.456205	0.452242	0.448283	0.44433	0.440382	0.436441	0.432505	0.428576	0.424655
0.2	0.42074	0.416834	0.412936	0.409046	0.405165	0.401294	0.397432	0.39358	0.389739	0.385908
0.3	0.382089	0.378281	0.374484	0.3707	0.366928	0.363169	0.359424	0.355691	0.351973	0.348268
0.4	0.344578	0.340903	0.337243	0.333598	0.329969	0.326355	0.322758	0.319178	0.315614	0.312067
0.5	0.308538	0.305026	0.301532	0.298056	0.294598	0.29116	0.28774	0.284339	0.280957	0.277595
0.6	0.274253	0.270931	0.267629	0.264347	0.261086	0.257846	0.254627	0.251429	0.248252	0.245097
0.7	0.241964	0.238852	0.235762	0.232695	0.22965	0.226627	0.223627	0.22065	0.217695	0.214764
0.8	0.211855	0.20897	0.206108	0.203269	0.200454	0.197662	0.194894	0.19215	0.18943	0.186733
0.9	0.18406	0.181411	0.178786	0.176186	0.173609	0.171056	0.168528	0.166023	0.163543	0.161087
1	0.158655	0.156248	0.153864	0.151505	0.14917	0.146859	0.144572	0.14231	0.140071	0.137857
1.1	0.135666	0.1335	0.131357	0.129238	0.127143	0.125072	0.123024	0.121001	0.119	0.117023
1.2	0.11507	0.11314	0.111233	0.109349	0.107488	0.10565	0.103835	0.102042	0.100273	0.098525
1.3	0.096801	0.095098	0.093418	0.091759	0.090123	0.088508	0.086915	0.085344	0.083793	0.082264
1.4	0.080757	0.07927	0.077804	0.076359	0.074934	0.073529	0.072145	0.070781	0.069437	0.068112
1.5	0.066807	0.065522	0.064256	0.063008	0.06178	0.060571	0.05938	0.058208	0.057053	0.055917
1.6	0.054799	0.053699	0.052616	0.051551	0.050503	0.049471	0.048457	0.04746	0.046479	0.045514
1.7	0.044565	0.043633	0.042716	0.041815	0.040929	0.040059	0.039204	0.038364	0.037538	0.036727
1.8	0.03593	0.035148	0.034379	0.033625	0.032884	0.032157	0.031443	0.030742	0.030054	0.029379
1.9	0.028716	0.028067	0.027429	0.026803	0.02619	0.025588	0.024998	0.024419	0.023852	0.023295

x	0	0.01	0.02	0.03	0.04	0.05	0.06	0.07	0.08	0.09
2	0.02275	0.022216	0.021692	0.021178	0.020675	0.020182	0.019699	0.019226	0.018763	0.018309
2.1	0.017864	0.017429	0.017003	0.016586	0.016177	0.015778	0.015386	0.015003	0.014629	0.014262
2.2	0.013903	0.013553	0.013209	0.012874	0.012545	0.012224	0.011911	0.011604	0.011304	0.011011
2.3	0.010724	0.010444	0.01017	0.009903	0.009642	0.009387	0.009137	0.008894	0.008656	0.008424
2.4	0.008198	0.007976	0.00776	0.007549	0.007344	0.007143	0.006947	0.006756	0.006569	0.006387
2.5	0.00621	0.006037	0.005868	0.005703	0.005543	0.005386	0.005234	0.005085	0.00494	0.004799
2.6	0.004661	0.004527	0.004397	0.004269	0.004145	0.004025	0.003907	0.003793	0.003681	0.003573
2.7	0.003467	0.003364	0.003264	0.003167	0.003072	0.00298	0.00289	0.002803	0.002718	0.002635
2.8	0.002555	0.002477	0.002401	0.002327	0.002256	0.002186	0.002118	0.002052	0.001988	0.001926
2.9	0.001866	0.001807	0.00175	0.001695	0.001641	0.001589	0.001538	0.001489	0.001441	0.001395
3	0.00135	0.001306	0.001264	0.001223	0.001183	0.001144	0.001107	0.00107	0.001035	0.001001
3.1	0.000968	0.000936	0.000904	0.000874	0.000845	0.000816	0.000789	0.000762	0.000736	0.000711
3.2	0.000687	0.000664	0.000641	0.000619	0.000598	0.000577	0.000557	0.000538	0.000519	0.000501
3.3	0.000483	0.000467	0.00045	0.000434	0.000419	0.000404	0.00039	0.000376	0.000362	0.00035
3.4	0.000337	0.000325	0.000313	0.000302	0.000291	0.00028	0.00027	0.00026	0.000251	0.000242
3.5	0.000233	0.000224	0.000216	0.000208	0.0002	0.000193	0.000185	0.000179	0.000172	0.000165
3.6	0.000159	0.000153	0.000147	0.000142	0.000136	0.000131	0.000126	0.000121	0.000117	0.000112
3.7	0.000108	0.000104	0.0001	0.000096	0.000092	0.000088	0.000085	0.000082	0.000078	0.000075
3.8	0.000072	0.00007	0.000067	0.000064	0.000062	0.000059	0.000057	0.000054	0.000052	0.00005
3.9	0.000048	0.000046	0.000044	0.000042	0.000041	0.000039	0.000037	0.000036	0.000034	0.000033

Appendix 3. Chi-Square Distribution

Upper tail probabilities for the Chi-square distribution are shown. For larger degrees of freedom, n, the distribution may be approximated as a normal distribution with

$$z = \frac{\left(\chi^2/n\right)^{1/3} - (1 - 2/(9n))}{(2/(9n))^{1/2}}$$

χ^2	$n = 1$	$n = 2$	$n = 3$	$n = 4$	$n = 5$
0.5	0.479500	0.778801	0.918891	0.973501	0.992123
1	0.317311	0.606531	0.801252	0.909796	0.962566
1.5	0.220671	0.472367	0.682270	0.826641	0.913070
2	0.157299	0.367879	0.572407	0.735759	0.849145
2.5	0.113846	0.286505	0.475291	0.644636	0.776495
3	0.083264	0.223130	0.391625	0.557825	0.699986
3.5	0.061369	0.173774	0.320762	0.477878	0.623387
4	0.045500	0.135335	0.261464	0.406006	0.549416
4.5	0.033895	0.105399	0.212290	0.342547	0.479883
5	0.025347	0.082085	0.171797	0.287297	0.415880
5.5	0.019016	0.063928	0.138639	0.239729	0.357946
6	0.014306	0.049787	0.111610	0.199148	0.306219
6.5	0.010787	0.038774	0.089663	0.164790	0.260559
7	0.008151	0.030197	0.071898	0.135888	0.220640
7.5	0.006170	0.023518	0.057559	0.111709	0.186030
8	0.004678	0.018316	0.046012	0.091578	0.156236
8.5	0.003552	0.014264	0.036733	0.074887	0.130748
9	0.002700	0.011109	0.029291	0.061099	0.109064
9.5	0.002055	0.008652	0.023331	0.049747	0.090708
10	0.001566	0.006738	0.018566	0.040428	0.075235
10.5	0.001194	0.005248	0.014761	0.032797	0.062246
11	0.000911	0.004087	0.011726	0.026564	0.051380

χ^2	$n = 1$	$n = 2$	$n = 3$	$n = 4$	$n = 5$
11.5	0.000696	0.003183	0.009308	0.021484	0.042320
12	0.000532	0.002479	0.007383	0.017351	0.034788
12.5	0.000407	0.001930	0.005853	0.013996	0.028543
13	0.000312	0.001503	0.004637	0.011276	0.023379
13.5	0.000239	0.001171	0.003671	0.009074	0.019118
14	0.000183	0.000912	0.002905	0.007295	0.015609
14.5	0.000140	0.000710	0.002298	0.005859	0.012727
15	0.000108	0.000553	0.001817	0.004701	0.010362
15.5	0.000083	0.000431	0.001436	0.003769	0.008427
16	0.000063	0.000335	0.001134	0.003019	0.006844
16.5	0.000049	0.000261	0.000895	0.002417	0.005553
17	0.000037	0.000203	0.000707	0.001933	0.004500
17.5	0.000029	0.000158	0.000558	0.001545	0.003643
18	0.000022	0.000123	0.000440	0.001234	0.002946
18.5	0.000017	0.000096	0.000347	0.000985	0.002381
19	0.000013	0.000075	0.000273	0.000786	0.001922
19.5	0.000010	0.000058	0.000215	0.000627	0.001551
20	0.000008	0.000045	0.000170	0.000499	0.001250
20.5	0.000006	0.000035	0.000134	0.000398	0.001007
21	0.000005	0.000028	0.000105	0.000317	0.000810
21.5	0.000004	0.000021	0.000083	0.000252	0.000651
22	0.000003	0.000017	0.000065	0.000200	0.000524
22.5	0.000002	0.000013	0.000051	0.000159	0.000421
23	0.000002	0.000010	0.000040	0.000127	0.000338
23.5	0.000001	0.000008	0.000032	0.000101	0.000271
24		0.000006	0.000025	0.000080	0.000217
24.5		0.000005	0.000020	0.000063	0.000174
25		0.000004	0.000015	0.000050	0.000139

χ^2	$n = 6$	$n = 7$	$n = 8$	$n = 9$	$n = 10$
5.0	0.543813				
6.0	0.423190	0.539749			
7.0	0.320847	0.428880	0.536633		
8.0	0.238103	0.332594	0.433470	0.534146	
9.0	0.173578	0.252656	0.342296	0.437274	0.532104
10.0	0.124652	0.188574	0.265026	0.350485	0.440493
11.0	0.088376	0.138619	0.201699	0.275709	0.357518
12.0	0.061969	0.100559	0.151204	0.213309	0.285057
13.0	0.043036	0.072108	0.111850	0.162606	0.223672
14.0	0.029636	0.051181	0.081765	0.122325	0.172992
15.0	0.020257	0.035999	0.059145	0.090936	0.132062
16.0	0.013754	0.025116	0.042380	0.066882	0.099632
17.0	0.009283	0.017396	0.030109	0.048716	0.074364
18.0	0.006232	0.011970	0.021226	0.035174	0.054964
19.0	0.004164	0.008187	0.014860	0.025193	0.040263
20.0	0.002769	0.005570	0.010336	0.017912	0.029253
21.0	0.001835	0.003770	0.007147	0.012650	0.021094
22.0	0.001211	0.002540	0.004916	0.008879	0.015105
23.0	0.000796	0.001705	0.003364	0.006196	0.010747
24.0	0.000522	0.001139	0.002292	0.004301	0.007600
25.0	0.000341	0.000759	0.001555	0.002971	0.005346
26.0	0.000223	0.000504	0.001050	0.002043	0.003740
27.0	0.000145	0.000333	0.000707	0.001399	0.002604
28.0	0.000094	0.000220	0.000474	0.000954	0.001805
29.0	0.000061	0.000145	0.000317	0.000648	0.001246
30.0	0.000039	0.000095	0.000211	0.000439	0.000857

χ^2	$n = 6$	$n = 7$	$n = 8$	$n = 9$	$n = 10$
31.0	0.000025	0.000062	0.000141	0.000296	0.000587
32.0	0.000016	0.000041	0.000093	0.000199	0.000400
33.0	0.000010	0.000026	0.000062	0.000134	0.000272
34.0	0.000007	0.000017	0.000041	0.000089	0.000185
35.0	0.000004	0.000011	0.000027	0.000060	0.000125
36.0	0.000003	0.000007	0.000018	0.000040	0.000084
37.0	0.000002	0.000005	0.000012	0.000026	0.000057
38.0	0.000001	0.000003	0.000008	0.000017	0.000038
39.0		0.000002	0.000005	0.000012	0.000025
40.0		0.000001	0.000003	0.000008	0.000017

χ^2	$n = 11$	$n = 12$	$n = 13$	$n = 14$	$n = 15$
10.0	0.530387	0.615961	0.693935	0.762183	0.819740
11.0	0.443263	0.528919	0.610818	0.686036	0.752594
12.0	0.363643	0.445680	0.527644	0.606303	0.679029
13.0	0.293325	0.369041	0.447812	0.526524	0.602298
14.0	0.232994	0.300708	0.373844	0.449711	0.525529
15.0	0.182497	0.241436	0.307353	0.378155	0.451417
16.0	0.141131	0.191236	0.249130	0.313374	0.382052
17.0	0.107876	0.149597	0.199304	0.256178	0.318864
18.0	0.081581	0.115691	0.157519	0.206781	0.262666
19.0	0.061094	0.088528	0.123104	0.164949	0.213734
20.0	0.045341	0.067086	0.095210	0.130141	0.171933
21.0	0.033371	0.050380	0.072929	0.101633	0.136829
22.0	0.024373	0.037520	0.055362	0.078614	0.107804
23.0	0.017675	0.027726	0.041676	0.060270	0.084140
24.0	0.012733	0.020341	0.031130	0.045822	0.065093
25.0	0.009117	0.014823	0.023084	0.034567	0.049943
26.0	0.006490	0.010734	0.017001	0.025887	0.038023
27.0	0.004595	0.007727	0.012441	0.019254	0.028736
28.0	0.003237	0.005532	0.009050	0.014228	0.021569
29.0	0.002270	0.003940	0.006546	0.010450	0.016085
30.0	0.001585	0.002792	0.004710	0.007632	0.011921
31.0	0.001102	0.001970	0.003372	0.005544	0.008785
32.0	0.000763	0.001384	0.002402	0.004006	0.006438
33.0	0.000526	0.000968	0.001704	0.002881	0.004694
34.0	0.000362	0.000675	0.001204	0.002062	0.003405

χ^2	$n = 11$	$n = 12$	$n = 13$	$n = 14$	$n = 15$
35.0	0.000248	0.000468	0.000847	0.001470	0.002459
36.0	0.000169	0.000324	0.000593	0.001043	0.001768
37.0	0.000115	0.000223	0.000414	0.000738	0.001266
38.0	0.000078	0.000154	0.000288	0.000520	0.000902
39.0	0.000053	0.000105	0.000200	0.000365	0.000641
40.0	0.000036	0.000072	0.000138	0.000255	0.000453
41.0	0.000024	0.000049	0.000095	0.000178	0.000320
42.0	0.000016	0.000033	0.000065	0.000124	0.000225
43.0	0.000011	0.000023	0.000045	0.000086	0.000157
44.0	0.000007	0.000015	0.000031	0.000059	0.000110
45.0	0.000005	0.000010	0.000021	0.000041	0.000077
46.0	0.000003	0.000007	0.000014	0.000028	0.000053
47.0	0.000002	0.000005	0.000010	0.000019	0.000037
48.0	0.000001	0.000003	0.000007	0.000013	0.000025

χ^2	$n = 16$	$n = 17$	$n = 18$	$n = 19$	$n = 20$
15.0	0.524639	0.595482	0.661967	0.722597	0.776408
16.0	0.452961	0.523835	0.592547	0.657278	0.716624
17.0	0.385597	0.454366	0.523105	0.589868	0.652974
18.0	0.323897	0.388841	0.455653	0.522438	0.587408
19.0	0.268663	0.328532	0.391823	0.456836	0.521826
20.0	0.220221	0.274229	0.332820	0.394578	0.457930
21.0	0.178511	0.226290	0.279413	0.336801	0.397133
22.0	0.143192	0.184719	0.231985	0.284256	0.340511
23.0	0.113735	0.149251	0.190590	0.237342	0.288795
24.0	0.089504	0.119435	0.155028	0.196152	0.242392
25.0	0.069825	0.094710	0.124916	0.160542	0.201431
26.0	0.054028	0.074461	0.099758	0.130189	0.165812
27.0	0.041483	0.058068	0.078995	0.104653	0.135264
28.0	0.031620	0.044938	0.062055	0.083429	0.109399
29.0	0.023936	0.034526	0.048379	0.065985	0.087759
30.0	0.018002	0.026345	0.037446	0.051798	0.069854
31.0	0.013456	0.019972	0.028787	0.040373	0.055190
32.0	0.010000	0.015048	0.021987	0.031255	0.043298
33.0	0.007390	0.011272	0.016690	0.024040	0.033741
34.0	0.005433	0.008396	0.012596	0.018378	0.026125
35.0	0.003974	0.006221	0.009452	0.013967	0.020104
36.0	0.002893	0.004587	0.007056	0.010556	0.015381
37.0	0.002097	0.003365	0.005241	0.007935	0.011702
38.0	0.001513	0.002458	0.003873	0.005935	0.008856
39.0	0.001088	0.001787	0.002850	0.004417	0.006667
40.0	0.000779	0.001294	0.002087	0.003272	0.004995

χ^2	$n = 16$	$n = 17$	$n = 18$	$n = 19$	$n = 20$
41.0	0.000555	0.000933	0.001522	0.002413	0.003725
42.0	0.000395	0.000671	0.001106	0.001772	0.002766
43.0	0.000279	0.000480	0.000800	0.001296	0.002044
44.0	0.000197	0.000343	0.000577	0.000944	0.001505
45.0	0.000139	0.000244	0.000414	0.000685	0.001103
46.0	0.000097	0.000173	0.000297	0.000496	0.000806
47.0	0.000068	0.000122	0.000212	0.000357	0.000587
48.0	0.000047	0.000086	0.000151	0.000257	0.000425
49.0	0.000033	0.000060	0.000107	0.000184	0.000307
50.0	0.000023	0.000042	0.000075	0.000131	0.000221
51.0	0.000016	0.000030	0.000053	0.000093	0.000159
52.0	0.000011	0.000021	0.000037	0.000066	0.000114
53.0	0.000008	0.000014	0.000026	0.000047	0.000081
54.0	0.000005	0.000010	0.000018	0.000033	0.000058
55.0	0.000004	0.000007	0.000013	0.000023	0.000041

Appendix 4. Wilcoxon Rank Sum Distribution

The upper tail of the distribution of the one-sided Wilcoxon Rank Sum statistic is shown. For values in the lower tail, enter the table with the value $W = n(m+n+1) - W_x$. For a two-sided test, simply double the P-value in the table.

$$n = 3$$

W	$m = 3$	$m = 4$	$m = 5$	$m = 6$	$m = 7$	$m = 8$
11	0.50000					
12	0.35000	0.57143				
13	0.20000	0.42857				
14	0.10000	0.31429	0.50000			
15	0.05000	0.20000	0.39286	0.54762		
16		0.11429	0.28571	0.45238		
17		0.05714	0.19643	0.35714	0.50000	
18		0.02857	0.12500	0.27381	0.41667	0.53939
19			0.07143	0.19048	0.33333	0.46061
20			0.03571	0.13095	0.25833	0.38788
21			0.01786	0.08333	0.19167	0.31515
22				0.04762	0.13333	0.24848
23				0.02381	0.09167	0.18788
24				0.01190	0.05833	0.13939
25					0.03333	0.09697
26					0.01667	0.06667
27					0.00833	0.04242
28						0.02424
29						0.01212
30						0.00606

$$n = 3$$

W	m = 9	m = 10
20	0.50000	
21	0.43182	0.53147
22	0.36364	0.46853
23	0.30000	0.40559
24	0.24091	0.34615
25	0.18636	0.28671
26	0.14091	0.23427
27	0.10455	0.18531
28	0.07273	0.14336
29	0.05000	0.10839
30	0.03182	0.08042
31	0.01818	0.05594
32	0.00909	0.03846
33	0.00455	0.02448
34		0.01399
35		0.00699
36		0.00350

$n = 4$

W	$m = 4$	$m = 5$	$m = 6$	$m = 7$	$m = 8$	$m = 9$	$m = 10$
18	0.55714						
19	0.44286						
20	0.34286	0.54762					
21	0.24286	0.45238					
22	0.17143	0.36508	0.54286				
23	0.10000	0.27778	0.45714				
24	0.05714	0.20635	0.38095	0.53636			
25	0.02857	0.14286	0.30476	0.46364			
26	0.01429	0.09524	0.23810	0.39394	0.53333		
27		0.05556	0.17619	0.32424	0.46667		
28		0.03175	0.12857	0.26364	0.40404	0.53007	
29		0.01587	0.08571	0.20606	0.34141	0.46993	
30		0.00794	0.05714	0.15758	0.28485	0.41259	0.52747
31			0.03333	0.11515	0.23030	0.35524	0.47253
32			0.01905	0.08182	0.18384	0.30210	0.41958
33			0.00952	0.05455	0.14141	0.25175	0.36663
34			0.00476	0.03636	0.10707	0.20699	0.31768
35				0.02121	0.07677	0.16503	0.26973
36				0.01212	0.05455	0.13007	0.22677
37				0.00606	0.03636	0.09930	0.18681
38				0.00303	0.02424	0.07413	0.15185
39					0.01414	0.05315	0.11988
40					0.00808	0.03776	0.09391
41					0.00404	0.02517	0.07093
42					0.00202	0.01678	0.05295
43						0.00979	0.03796
44						0.00559	0.02697
45						0.00280	0.01798
46						0.00140	0.01199

$n = 4$

W	$m = 10$
47	0.00699
48	0.00400
49	0.00200
50	0.00100

$n = 5$

W	$m = 5$	$m = 6$	$m = 7$	$m = 8$	$m = 9$	$m = 10$
28	0.50000					
29	0.42063					
30	0.34524	0.53463				
31	0.27381	0.46537				
32	0.21032	0.39610				
33	0.15476	0.33117	0.50000			
34	0.11111	0.26840	0.43813			
35	0.07540	0.21429	0.37753	0.52836		
36	0.04762	0.16450	0.31944	0.47164		
37	0.02778	0.12338	0.26515	0.41647		
38	0.01587	0.08874	0.21591	0.36208	0.50000	
39	0.00794	0.06277	0.17172	0.31080	0.44905	
40	0.00397	0.04113	0.13384	0.26185	0.39860	0.52348
41		0.02597	0.10101	0.21756	0.34965	0.47652
42		0.01515	0.07449	0.17716	0.30320	0.42957
43		0.00866	0.05303	0.14219	0.25924	0.38395
44		0.00433	0.03662	0.11111	0.21878	0.33933
45		0.00216	0.02399	0.08547	0.18182	0.29704
46			0.01515	0.06371	0.14885	0.25674
47			0.00884	0.04662	0.11988	0.21978
48			0.00505	0.03263	0.09491	0.18548
49			0.00253	0.02253	0.07343	0.15485
50			0.00126	0.01476	0.05594	0.12721
51				0.00932	0.04146	0.10323
52				0.00544	0.02997	0.08225
53				0.00311	0.02098	0.06460
54				0.00155	0.01449	0.04962
55				0.00078	0.00949	0.03763

$$n = 5$$

W	$m = 9$	$m = 10$
56	0.00599	0.02764
57	0.00350	0.01998
58	0.00200	0.01399
59	0.00100	0.00966
60	0.00050	0.00633
61		0.00400
62		0.00233
63		0.00133
64		0.00067
65		0.00033

$$n = 6$$

W	m = 6	m = 7	m = 8	m = 9	m = 10
39	0.53139				
40	0.46861				
41	0.40909				
42	0.34957	0.52739			
43	0.29437	0.47261			
44	0.24242	0.41783			
45	0.19697	0.36538	0.52514		
46	0.15476	0.31410	0.47486		
47	0.12013	0.26690	0.42591		
48	0.08983	0.22261	0.37729	0.52268	
49	0.06602	0.18298	0.33100	0.47732	
50	0.04654	0.14744	0.28638	0.43197	
51	0.03247	0.11713	0.24542	0.38781	0.52110
52	0.02056	0.09033	0.20679	0.34446	0.47890
53	0.01299	0.06876	0.17249	0.30350	0.43744
54	0.00758	0.05070	0.14119	0.26434	0.39623
55	0.00433	0.03671	0.11422	0.22797	0.35639
56	0.00216	0.02564	0.09058	0.19421	0.31768
57	0.00108	0.01748	0.07093	0.16384	0.28109
58		0.01107	0.05395	0.13606	0.24613
59		0.00699	0.04063	0.11189	0.21391
60		0.00408	0.02964	0.09051	0.18382
61		0.00233	0.02131	0.07233	0.15659
62		0.00117	0.01465	0.05674	0.13174
63		0.00058	0.00999	0.04396	0.10989
64			0.00633	0.03317	0.09028
65			0.00400	0.02478	0.07355

$$n = 6$$

W	$m = 8$	$m = 9$	$m = 10$
66	0.00233	0.01798	0.05894
67	0.00133	0.01279	0.04670
68	0.00067	0.00879	0.03634
69	0.00033	0.00599	0.02797
70		0.00380	0.02098
71		0.00240	0.01561
72		0.00140	0.01124
73		0.00080	0.00799
74		0.00040	0.00549
75		0.00020	0.00375
76			0.00237
77			0.00150
78			0.00087
79			0.00050
80			0.00025
81			0.00012

$$n = 7$$

W	m = 7	m = 8	m = 9	m = 10
53	0.500000			
54	0.450758			
55	0.402389			
56	0.355186	0.522455		
57	0.310023	0.477545		
58	0.267483	0.433256		
59	0.227855	0.389433		
60	0.191434	0.347164	0.500000	
61	0.158800	0.306294	0.459091	
62	0.129662	0.267910	0.418531	
63	0.104312	0.231702	0.378846	0.518871
64	0.082459	0.198446	0.340297	0.481129
65	0.064103	0.167832	0.303234	0.443387
66	0.048660	0.140482	0.268007	0.406263
67	0.036422	0.115929	0.234878	0.369807
68	0.026515	0.094639	0.203934	0.334533
69	0.018939	0.075991	0.175524	0.300442
70	0.013112	0.060295	0.149563	0.268100
71	0.008741	0.046931	0.126136	0.237351
72	0.005536	0.036053	0.105245	0.208659
73	0.003497	0.027040	0.086888	0.181921
74	0.002040	0.020047	0.070804	0.157394
75	0.001166	0.014452	0.057080	0.134924
76	0.000583	0.010256	0.045367	0.114768
77	0.000291	0.006993	0.035577	0.096617
78		0.004662	0.027448	0.080625
79		0.002953	0.020892	0.066536
80		0.001865	0.015559	0.054401

$$n = 7$$

W	$m = 8$	$m = 9$	$m = 10$
81	0.001088	0.011451	0.043912
82	0.000622	0.008217	0.035119
83	0.000311	0.005769	0.027664
84	0.000155	0.003934	0.021545
85		0.002622	0.016506
86		0.001661	0.012495
87		0.001049	0.009255
88		0.000612	0.006787
89		0.000350	0.004833
90		0.000175	0.003394
91		0.000087	0.002314
92			0.001543
93			0.000977
94			0.000617
95			0.000360
96			0.000206
97			0.000103
98			0.000051

$n = 8$

W	$m = 8$	$m = 9$	$m = 10$
68	0.520435		
69	0.479565		
70	0.439239		
71	0.399223		
72	0.360451	0.518717	
73	0.322688	0.481283	
74	0.286869	0.444179	
75	0.252681	0.407404	
76	0.220901	0.371493	0.517300
77	0.191142	0.336487	0.482700
78	0.164103	0.302921	0.448375
79	0.139316	0.270712	0.414279
80	0.117249	0.240354	0.380913
81	0.097436	0.211724	0.348233
82	0.080264	0.185191	0.316719
83	0.065190	0.160633	0.286302
84	0.052448	0.138297	0.257393
85	0.041492	0.117935	0.229878
86	0.032479	0.099794	0.204123
87	0.024942	0.083587	0.179967
88	0.018959	0.069395	0.157708
89	0.014064	0.056972	0.137141
90	0.010334	0.046360	0.118493
91	0.007382	0.037227	0.101536
92	0.005206	0.029617	0.086407
93	0.003497	0.023200	0.072855
94	0.002331	0.017976	0.060995

$n = 8$

W	$m = 8$	$m = 9$	$m = 10$
95	0.001476	0.013698	0.050551
96	0.000932	0.010325	0.041570
97	0.000544	0.007610	0.033800
98	0.000311	0.005553	0.027264
99	0.000155	0.003949	0.021710
100	0.000078	0.002756	0.017140
101		0.001851	0.013323
102		0.001234	0.010261
103		0.000782	0.007770
104		0.000494	0.005828
105		0.000288	0.004274
106		0.000165	0.003108
107		0.000082	0.002194
108		0.000041	0.001531
109			0.001028
110			0.000686
111			0.000434
112			0.000274
113			0.000160
114			0.000091
115			0.000046
116			0.000023

$$n = 9$$

W	$m = 9$	$m = 10$	W	$m = 9$	$m = 10$
86	0.500000		114	0.005306	0.026738
87	0.465714		115	0.003887	0.021737
88	0.431654		118	0.001378	0.011009
89	0.398087		119	0.000926	0.008606
90	0.365220	0.515880	120	0.000617	0.006636
91	0.333237	0.484120	121	0.000391	0.005066
92	0.302406	0.452413	122	0.000247	0.003810
93	0.272851	0.421053	123	0.000144	0.002836
94	0.244714	0.390093	124	0.000082	0.002068
95	0.218141	0.359848	125	0.000041	0.001494
96	0.193254	0.330360	126	0.000021	0.001050
97	0.170053	0.301890	127		0.000725
98	0.148663	0.274481	128		0.000487
99	0.129042	0.248349	129		0.000325
100	0.111209	0.223484	130		0.000206
101	0.095125	0.200091	131		0.000130
102	0.080749	0.178116	132		0.000076
103	0.067956	0.157689	133		0.000043
104	0.056746	0.138756	134		0.000022
105	0.046956	0.121403	135		0.000011
106	0.038503	0.105512			
107	0.031263	0.091158			
108	0.025154	0.078200			
109	0.019992	0.066650			
110	0.015734	0.056377			
111	0.012217	0.047360			
112	0.009379	0.039447			
113	0.007096	0.032627			

$$n = 10$$

W	$m = 10$	W	$m = 10$
105	0.514744	131	0.026213
106	0.485256	132	0.021629
107	0.455899	133	0.017731
108	0.426714	134	0.014403
109	0.397968	135	0.011615
110	0.369682	136	0.009272
111	0.342105	137	0.007345
112	0.315264	138	0.005748
113	0.289371	139	0.004465
114	0.264424	140	0.003421
115	0.240625	141	0.002598
116	0.217936	142	0.001943
117	0.196524	143	0.001440
118	0.176341	144	0.001045
119	0.157500	145	0.000752
120	0.139931	146	0.000525
121	0.123725	147	0.000363
122	0.108781	148	0.000244
123	0.095158	149	0.000162
124	0.082747	150	0.000103
125	0.071570	151	0.000065
126	0.061503	152	0.000038
127	0.052561	153	0.000022
128	0.044605	154	0.000011
129	0.037628	155	0.000005
130	0.031506		

Appendix 5. Wilcoxon Signed Rank Distribution

The lower tail of the distribution of the statistic is given below.

W	$n = 4$	$n = 5$	$n = 6$	$n = 7$	$n = 8$
0	0.06250	0.03125	0.01563	0.00781	0.00391
1	0.12500	0.06250	0.03125	0.01563	0.00781
2	0.18750	0.09375	0.04688	0.02344	0.01172
3	0.31250	0.15625	0.07813	0.03906	0.01953
4	0.43750	0.21875	0.10938	0.05469	0.02734
5	0.56250	0.31250	0.15625	0.07813	0.03906
6	0.68750	0.40625	0.21875	0.10938	0.05469
7	0.81250	0.50000	0.28125	0.14844	0.07422
8	0.87500	0.59375	0.34375	0.18750	0.09766
9	0.93750	0.68750	0.42188	0.23438	0.12500
10	1.00000	0.78125	0.50000	0.28906	0.15625
11		0.84375	0.57813	0.34375	0.19141
12		0.90625	0.65625	0.40625	0.23047
13		0.93750	0.71875	0.46875	0.27344
14		0.96875	0.78125	0.53125	0.32031
15		1.00000	0.84375	0.59375	0.37109
16			0.89063	0.65625	0.42188
17			0.92188	0.71094	0.47266
18			0.95313	0.76563	0.52734
19			0.96875	0.81250	0.57813
20			0.98438	0.85156	0.62891
21			1.00000	0.89063	0.67969
22				0.92188	0.72656
23				0.94531	0.76953

W	$n = 9$	$n = 10$	$n = 11$	$n = 12$	$n = 13$
0	0.00195	0.00098	0.00049	0.00024	0.00012
1	0.00391	0.00195	0.00098	0.00049	0.00024
2	0.00586	0.00293	0.00146	0.00073	0.00037
3	0.00977	0.00488	0.00244	0.00122	0.00061
4	0.01367	0.00684	0.00342	0.00171	0.00085
5	0.01953	0.00977	0.00488	0.00244	0.00122
6	0.02734	0.01367	0.00684	0.00342	0.00171
7	0.03711	0.01855	0.00928	0.00464	0.00232
8	0.04883	0.02441	0.01221	0.00610	0.00305
9	0.06445	0.03223	0.01611	0.00806	0.00403
10	0.08203	0.04199	0.02100	0.01050	0.00525
11	0.10156	0.05273	0.02686	0.01343	0.00671
12	0.12500	0.06543	0.03369	0.01709	0.00854
13	0.15039	0.08008	0.04150	0.02124	0.01074
14	0.17969	0.09668	0.05078	0.02612	0.01331
15	0.21289	0.11621	0.06152	0.03198	0.01636
16	0.24805	0.13770	0.07373	0.03857	0.01990
17	0.28516	0.16113	0.08740	0.04614	0.02393
18	0.32617	0.18750	0.10303	0.05493	0.02869
19	0.36719	0.21582	0.12012	0.06470	0.03406
20	0.41016	0.24609	0.13916	0.07568	0.04016
21	0.45508	0.27832	0.16016	0.08813	0.04712
22	0.50000	0.31250	0.18262	0.10181	0.05493
23		0.34766	0.20654	0.11670	0.06360
24		0.38477	0.23242	0.13306	0.07324
25		0.42285	0.25977	0.15063	0.08386

W	n = 9	n = 10	n = 11	n = 12	n = 13
26		0.46094	0.28857	0.16968	0.09546
27		0.50000	0.31885	0.19019	0.10815
28			0.35010	0.21191	0.12195
29			0.38232	0.23486	0.13672
30			0.41553	0.25928	0.15271
31			0.44922	0.28467	0.16980
32			0.48291	0.31104	0.18787
33			0.51709	0.33862	0.20715
34				0.36670	0.22742
35				0.39551	0.24866
36				0.42505	0.27087
37				0.45483	0.29395
38				0.48486	0.31775
39				0.51514	0.34241
40					0.36768
41					0.39343
42					0.41968
43					0.44629
44					0.47302
45					0.50000

Appendix 6. Kendall's Rank Correlation Distribution

The upper tail of the distribution is shown. For sample sizes larger than 8, the normal approximation to the distribution is quite accurate.

K	n = 4	n = 5	n = 6	n = 7	n = 8
0	0.625000	0.591667			0.547569
1			0.500000	0.500000	
2	0.375000	0.408333			0.452431
3			0.359722	0.386310	
4	0.166667	0.241667			0.359772
5			0.234722	0.280952	
6	0.041667	0.116667			0.274206
7			0.136111	0.190675	
8		0.041667			0.199380
9			0.068056	0.119444	
10		0.008333			0.137550
11			0.027778	0.068056	
12					0.089435
13			0.008333	0.034524	
14					0.054340
15			0.001389	0.015079	
16					0.030506
17				0.005357	
18					0.015575
19				0.001389	
20					0.007068
21				0.000198	

K	n = 4	n = 5	n = 6	n = 7	n = 8
22					0.002753
23					
24					0.000868
25					
26					0.000198
27					
28					0.000025

APPENDIX 7. MSTAT 5.5 USER MANUAL

INTRODUCTION

Mstat was developed to provide a simple approach to analyzing data using nonparametric statistical methods. This program grew out of a graduate course, *Statistical Problems in Genetics and Molecular Biology,* taught jointly by the Departments of Oncology and Genetics at the University of Wisconsin-Madison over the last 20 years. A hypertext version of the notes for the course is accessible from the program's help file.

Mstat was written in J (Version 6.02), an *Array Programming Language* developed by JSoftware, Inc. Windows, Macintosh OS X, and Linux versions of *Mstat* are distributed as standalone applications and require the appropriate J runtime executable (which is provided as part of the *Mstat* package). The Windows version should run on all versions of the operating system newer than Windows NT, and requires no additional software. The OS X and Linux versions require Java (version 1.4.2 or later). Other minor differences in the operation of the Mac and Linux versions are detailed below in *Mac/Linux Specifics*. Legacy versions of the program for Windows 9x and Macintosh OS9 are available from the website. As of version 5.2, both 64-bit and 32-bit versions of the software are available for Windows and Linux.

Version 5.5 is the fourteenth general release of *Mstat*. Major changes from version 4.x largely focused on the plotting functions. More plot types are available and increased control over the appearance of the plots should allow you to generate (near) publication quality graphs from your data. It is now also possible to produce power plots that show families of curves with differing power or distribution parameters. Finally, upgrading to version 6 of the J engine has greatly improved the speed and responsiveness of the program on OSX and Linux.

To be kept apprised of updates to *Mstat*, send an email to drinkwater@oncology.wisc.edu that includes the version you are using (available in the *About* box under the *Help* menu). You can also check the website at http://mcardle.oncology.wisc.edu/mstat.

TUTORIAL

This tutorial will work through a short *Mstat* session to familiarize you with the operation of the program. A more comprehensive reference section follows.

In the examples below, you have tumor multiplicity data for two groups of animals (heterozygous or homozygous for a particular locus) and want to test the hypothesis that the genotypes differ in their cancer risk. The data are:

homozygous	0 0 0 4 6 7 20 1 19 14 8 19 5 16 26 3 2
	16 1 2 1 0 12 12 1 0 0 0 6 5 0 5 0 0 5
	1 0 2 0 11 6 0 3 0 6 0
heterozygous	5 10 28 5 27 0 19 10 26 1 53 2 49 38 21
	15 25 18 1 71 1 15 18 3 44 2 3 74 52 37 7
	12 26 58 9 2 2 12 35 0 18 2 1 0 3 6 3 6
	28 2

We will also import similar data from an Excel spreadsheet that was saved as a "CSV" (comma-separated variable) file.

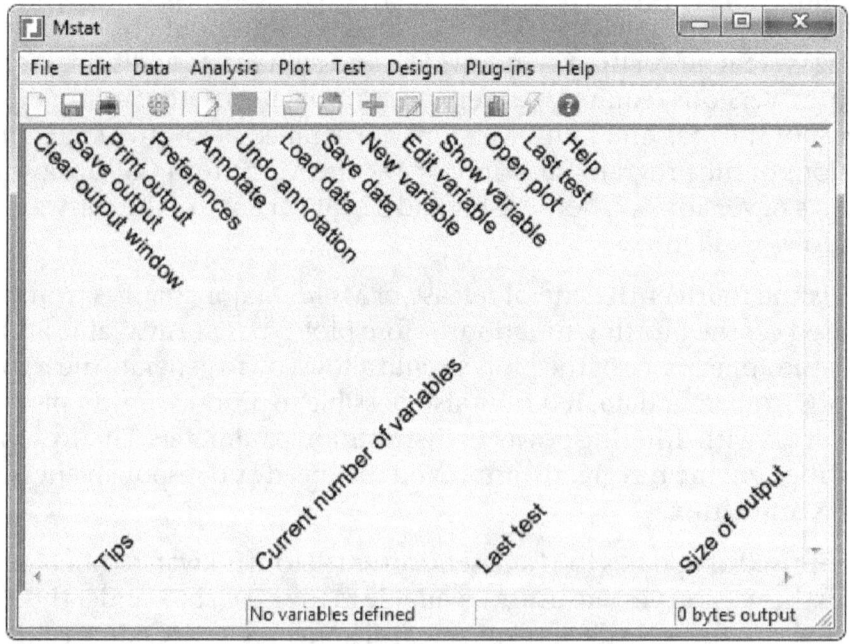

Starting the program.

Start the program by clicking on the *Mstat* entry in Start Programs (Win) or double-clicking the *Mstat* icon (Mac). The main program window (see above) consists of a menu bar and toolbar for choosing program functions, an output window for displaying your results, and a statusbar that displays information about the current session as well as brief explanations of the menu and toolbar functions (place the mouse over a toolbar button to see the tip in the statusbar). Each toolbar button is equivalent to a menu entry, except for the *Last test* button, which is assigned to the most recently chosen item from the *Analysis*, *Test*, or *Design* menus.

Entering and editing data.

The three data types in *Mstat* are stored as arrays (lists) of numbers or characters or as tables (Variables, Indicators, and Tables, respectively). An Indicator stores a list of non-numeric values that can be used to subdivide a regular variable into various groups (see example below). It could also be used to store a list of labels for a bar graph.

The name for an *Mstat* variable can be of any length, must start with a letter, and consists of a sequence of letters, numeric digits, or the underscore character (no spaces, punctuation marks, or other special characters; the name cannot contain a double underscore or end in an underscore). Variable names are case-sensitive, *i.e.*, "Mutant", "mutant", and "MuTaNt" all refer to distinct variables. The same name can be used simultaneously for each of the three data types (at the cost of some confusion), but within each type, every variable name must be unique. You should try to choose variable names that are meaningful to you. *Mstat* variables may be stored on disk as text files (see below) so all of the data entered in an *Mstat* session may be reloaded into the program for later use.

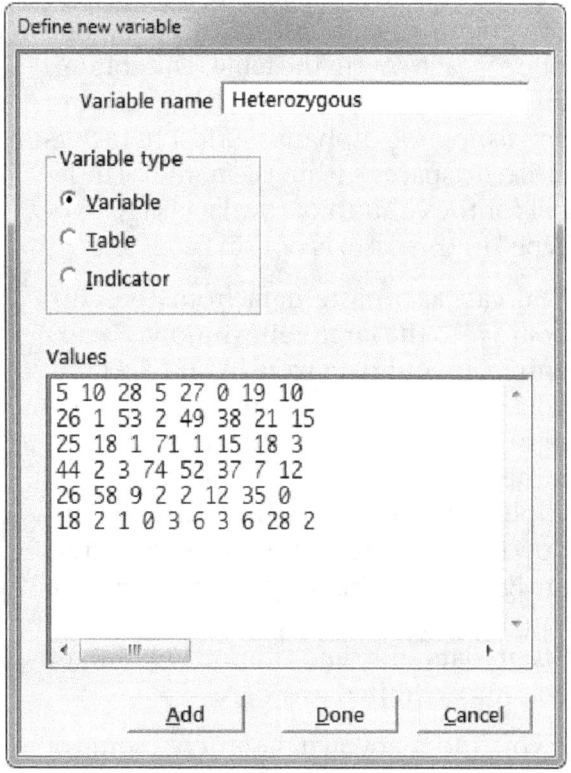

In order to define a new variable, choose *New* from the *Data* menu, or click on the *New variable* button on the toolbar. You will then see the following dialog box at right.

Enter your new variable name (in this case Heterozygous) in the upper window, select the appropriate variable type from among the radiobuttons, and tab to the larger window to enter your data. You should enter numbers in simple (*e.g.*, 1 -3.5 2.0215) or exponential (*e.g.*, 3.2e-5) format separated by spaces or carriage-returns. When you have finished entering the data, click on the *Add* button (if you wish to define additional variables) or the *Done* button. A new feature added in version 3.2 allows the use of J notation to define the data (see Reference section). You will most often use this feature for entering repeated values. For example, the six values of "2" could be specified as (6#2) [the parentheses aren't required but are advisable]. If the edit window contains non-numeric data (or data that doesn't evaluate to a list of numbers in J), you will see an error message, and you'll be given the opportunity to edit the data. If you chose a variable name that is already defined, you will also get an error message and the chance to enter a new name. After *Add*ing the data, the dialog box will be cleared, and you can define an additional variable. Do that to define the Homozygous variable.

Both the Heterozygous and Homozygous variables are simple one-dimensional data arrays. You can also enter data in a tabular form that is appropriate for contingency tables. Define a new variable and select the *Table* radiobutton. You can enter the data as a table in the edit box with appropriate column and row headings. Entry is free form (*i.e.*, the number of spaces separating the entries doesn't matter), but you must have a line with

the column headings, followed by one line for each row in the table. The column and row headings must each be one word consisting of alphanumeric characters (with no spaces within the name). The label for the column of row labels ("Genotype" in this case) is optional.

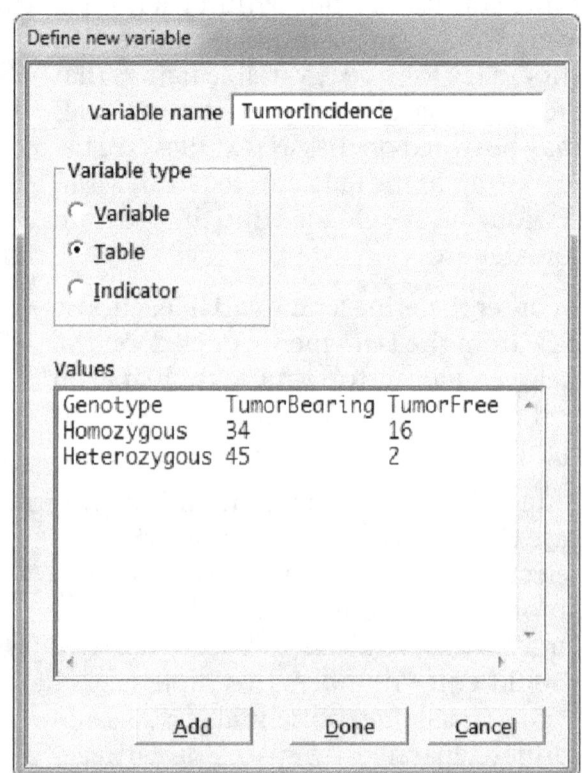

You can also paste data from the clipboard into the large edit window. For example, if your data were in an Excel file, you could open the spreadsheet, highlight the column or row of cells that contained the desired data, copy it to the clipboard, and paste it into the edit window (tabs or other white space characters are ignored). Other ways of bringing data into the program include loading a saved *Mstat* data file and importing tab or comma-delimited text files.

If you find that you have entered some of the data incorrectly (*e.g.*, after you've used the *Show* function to print the data to the output window), you can edit the variable by choosing *Edit* from the *Data* menu or by clicking the *Edit data* button on the toolbar. You will get the following dialog box below.

Select the appropriate variable type, choose the name of the variable to be edited from the list box (highlight the desired name and double-click or press enter). The data associated with that variable will be displayed for editing in the window below. If you want to change the name of the variable, select the *Edit variable name* checkbox to enable the variable name edit box. When you have finished modifying the data (or variable name), press the *Change* or *Done* button. The dialog box will stay open to allow additional editing until *Done* is pressed.

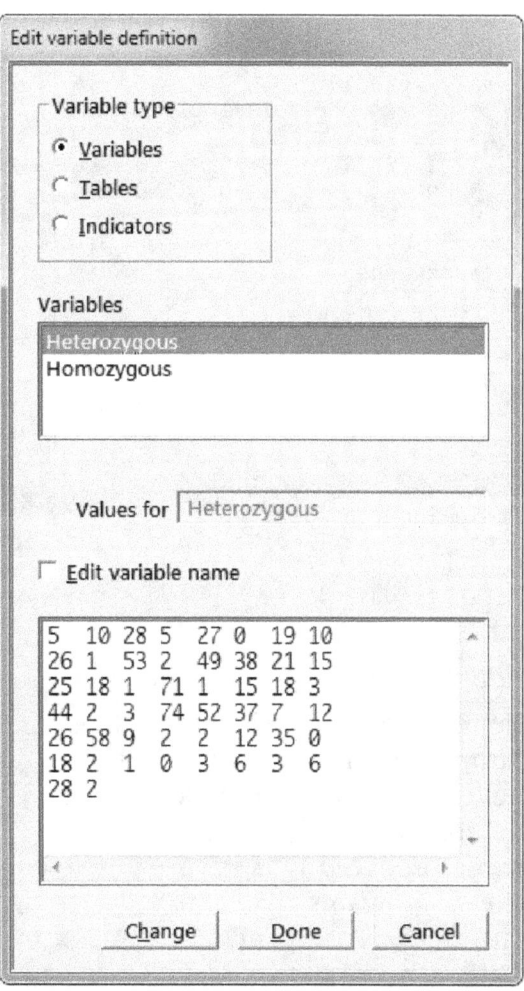

Show the data in the output window.

In order to make sure that you've correctly entered the data, print the variables to the output window by choosing *Show* from the *Data* menu or pressing the *Show data* button on the toolbar. Select the desired variable type, select (highlight and double-click or press *Add*) the variable(s) you want to show from the *Available* variables list and its name will move from the list box on the left to that on the right of the window. When you have selected all of the variables in the desired order, press *Done* to show the contents of the variables. If you want to print the contents of another variable type to the output window, you will need to reopen the dialog box.

After choosing the two available variables and then the table, you should see the following in the output window:

```
Homozygous
0    0    0    4    6    7   20  1   19  14  8
19   5   16   26  32   16   1  2    1   0
12  12    1    0   0    0    0  6    5   0
5    0    0    5   1    0    2  0   11   6   0
3    0    6    0

Heterozygous
5   10  28   5   27   0   19  10  26  1
53   2  49  38  21  15
25  18   1  71   1   15  18   3  44   2   3
74  52  37   7  12
26  58   9   2   2   12  35   0  18   2   1
0    3   6   3   6
28   2
```

```
Table TumorIncidence
Genotype          TumorBearing    TumorFree
Homozygous             34             16
Heterozygous           45              3
```

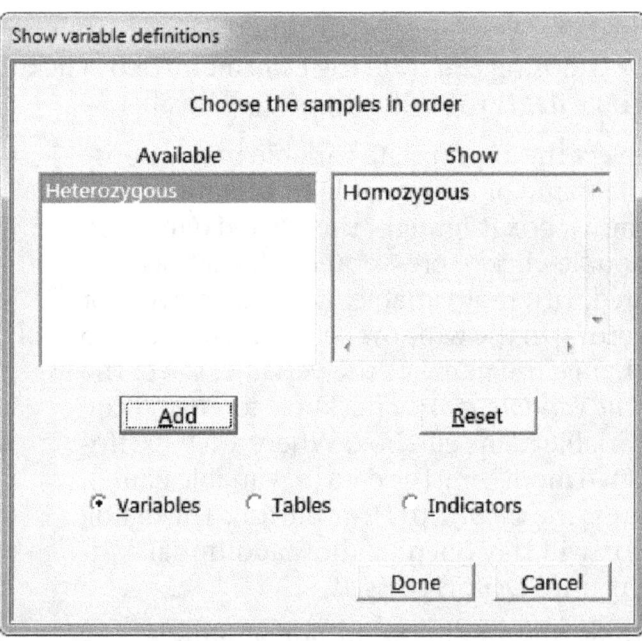

Importing data.

You can import data into an *Mstat* session from a tab-delimited or comma-delimited text file, such as those produced by spread-sheet programs like Microsoft Excel or OpenOffice Calc. Choose *Import data* from the *File* menu and select the file, tutorial.csv, from the file open dialog and you will get a dialog box as follows:

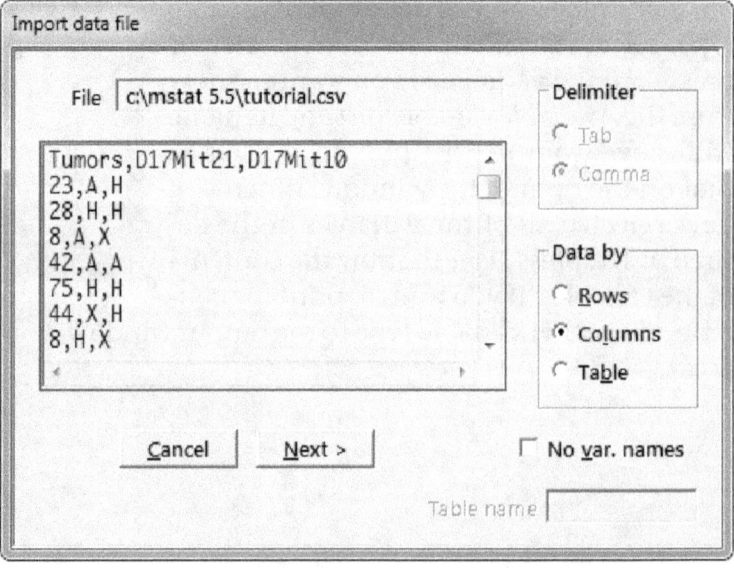

The file name appears in the edit box at the top of the dialog and the first lines of the file appear in the edit window below it. Based on the contents of the file, the appropriate radiobutton for the delimiter (comma in this case) is selected. The set of radiobuttons in the *Data by* group allow you to specify whether the data in the file should be read by rows or columns, or should be converted into a single table variable. If you choose *Table* you need to enter a *Table name*. If the first row (for column format), or first column (for row format) does not contain the names of the variables, check the *No var. names* box and you will be prompted for variable names. When you've made the appropriate choices, press the *Next* button to bring up the following dialog:

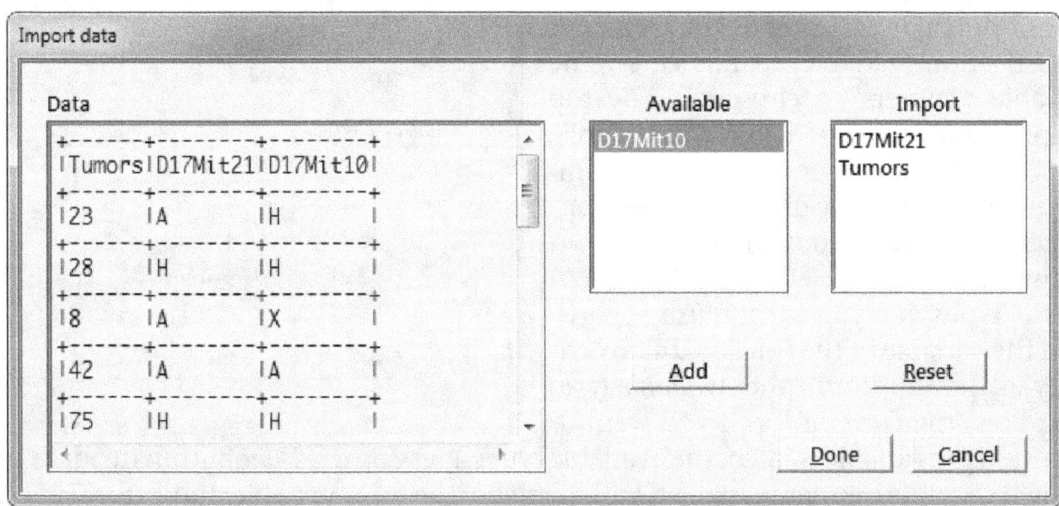

The edit box at the left shows the parsed data. Note that the first column contains numeric data, but the second two contain non-numeric data. These latter two columns would be converted to indicator variables (see below) while the former would be saved as a regular variable. The available variables are listed in the first listbox. You can choose to import any or all of them by double-clicking the variable name(s) or selecting one or more names and pressing *Add*. When all of the desired variables are listed in the *Import* listbox, press *Done*.

Indicator variables.

Indicator variables allow you to partition a regular variable (or another indicator variable) into subgroups based on the value of the indicator variable. Both variables must have the same number of values. In our example above, we imported a set of numeric observations (Tumors) and a single indicator variable (D17Mit21), which contains the genotype at a particular locus for each observation represented in the Tumors variable. Although, in this case, each indicator is represented by a single character (A, H, or X), an indicator variable can contain any arbitrary data (for example, the entries could be "homozygous", "heterozygous", and "unknown"). Leading and trailing spaces in the data are removed during the import.

To subdivide a regular variable according to an indicator, choose *Classify* from the *Data* menu to get the following dialog box:

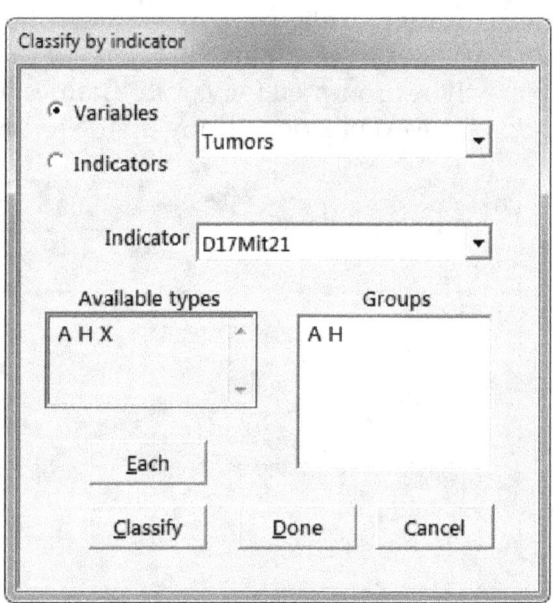

The radiobuttons allow you to select indicator or regular variables as the target for classification (variables in this case). The variable "Tumors" is chosen in the top dropbox and the desired indicator variable, "D17Mit21", is chosen from the one immediately below. The distinct entries contained in the indicator variable are shown in the edit box at the left of the dialog. Enter the types that you wish to use to partition the variable in the *Groups* edit box exactly as they appear in the *Available types* box. Press the *Each* button if you want to partition the variable by all of the available types. Pressing the *Done* button in our example will generate two new variables, with names of the form Variable_Indicator_Type. In our case, we will make two new variables, Tumors_D17Mit21_A and Tumors_D17Mit21_H, that divide the Tumors variable into two groups, those observations for which the associated type is A and those of type H. Showing the new variables to the output window gives

```
Tumors_D17Mit21_A
23 8   42 0   36 7   0   5   2   8   16 5   5   13 3   7
4   5   4   3   4   5   3   2   2   25 5   0   3   11 29

Tumors_D17Mit21_H
28 75 8   16 45 44 69 57 47 45 30 39 25 15 26 8
25 50 10 44 0   12 47 29
```

Describing data.

The analysis menu has several choices useful for describing your data, including tabulating the means, variances, and quantiles for several variables, or the sample distributions for one or more variables, as well as some simple data plots.

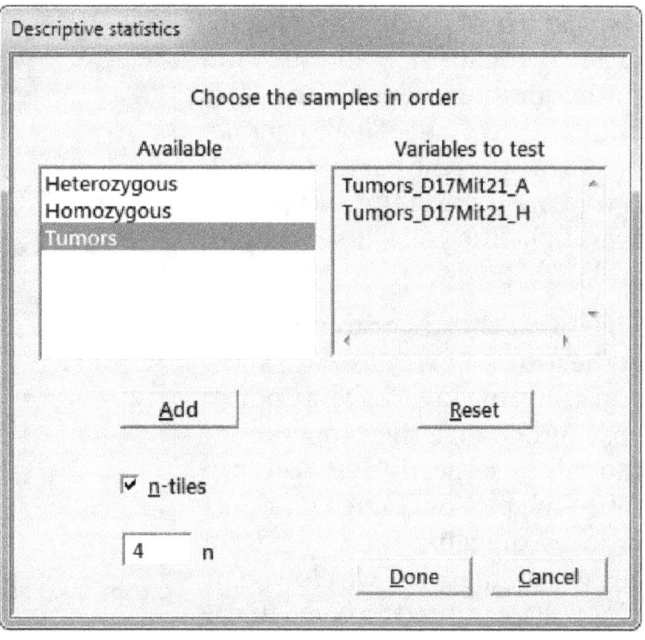

To display the means and standard deviations of some of your variables, choose *Descriptive* from the *Analysis* menu to obtain the following dialog box.

Choose the desired variables in the order that you want them to appear in the output table by double-clicking the name in the *Available* variables list or highlighting the name and pressing the *Add* button. *Reset* moves all of the variables back to the *Available* box. If you check the *n-tiles* box and enter 4 in the box immediately below it, the output table will also display the data values for the 1st, 2nd, and 3rd quartiles, as well as the minimum and maximum observations. (To show only the median, enter "2" in the box labeled *n*.) Press *Done* to display the output.

```
Descriptive statistics
Sample            N    Mean   Std. dev.   4-tile         Min   Max
Tumors_D17Mit21_A  31   9.194  10.73       3  5  9.5       0     42
Tumors_D17Mit21_H  24   33.08  19.82       15.5 29.5 46   0     75
```

Graphical plots of your data can often provide helpful insights and are obviously useful for explaining your results to other people. *Mstat* does a number of fairly simple plots, including histograms of sample distributions, a variety of bar graphs, survival plots, X-Y plots for bivariate data, regression analyses, power plots, and dot plots for comparing several sample distributions.

Choose *Dot plot* from the *Plot* menu to get the following dialog box at right.

Select both variables as described above for *Descriptive statistics* (note the similarity in the dialog boxes). If you want your plot to have an origin of 0 on the Y-axis, check the *Range includes 0* box. To display a bar indicating the median and first and third quartiles next to the data points, select the *Show quartiles* box. Note that the bar may partially obscure some of the data points. Press *Done* and you will see the plot at the left below.

The menu choices or four buttons at the top of the window will allow you to print, save, save as pdf or eps, and change the properties of the plot, respectively. You can resize the plot or change its aspect ratio by dragging the lower right corner of the plot window. The plot will be printed or saved in the

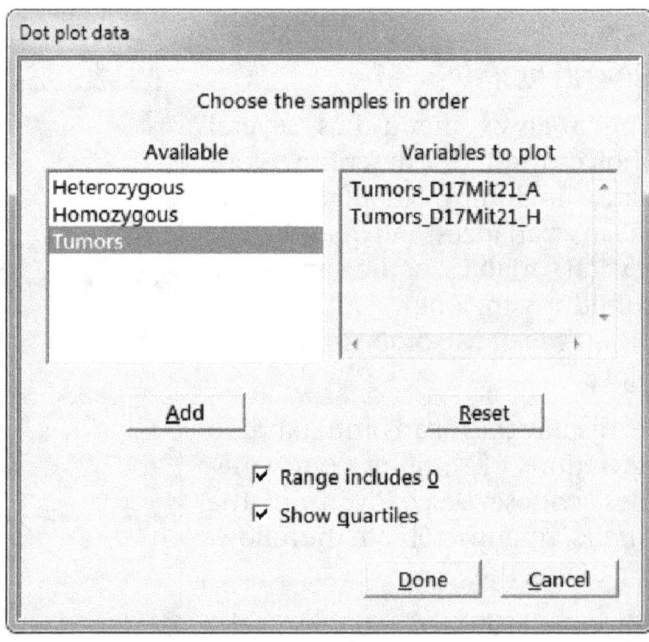

same shape and approximately the same size as it is shown on screen. Plots may also be saved as PDF or EPS files, which may be printed or edited in Adobe Illustrator, the open source Inkscape drawing program, or other applications.

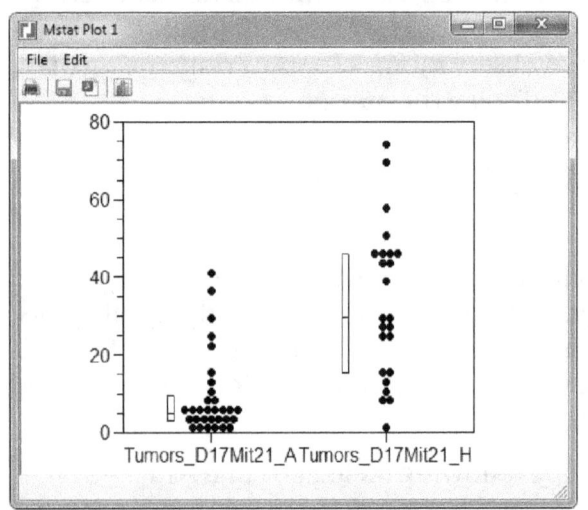

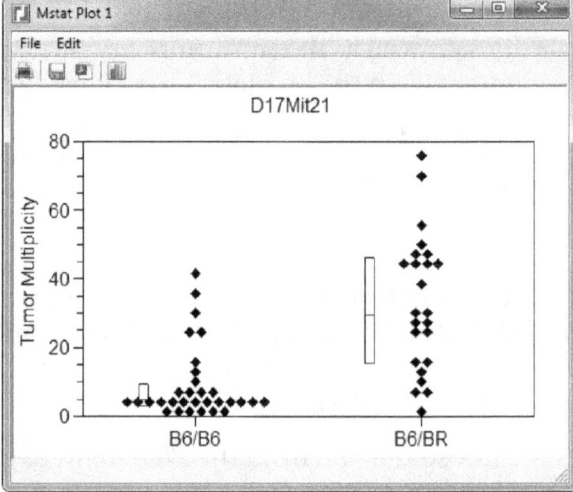

Press the *Modify plot* button (the right-most button) to get the dialog at right. The four tabs allow you to modify the size or text of the labels or captions; the ranges of the axes, tic size or tic interval; the shape, size, or color of the symbols; and the contents or position of the plot key. For our plot, change the *Group names* on the X axis to "B6/B6" and "B6/BR", enter the text "D17Mit21" in the title box, and add a Y-axis label (Tumor multiplicity). Change to the *Symbols* tab and use the dropdown boxes to change the *Color* to Red for each group and the *Marker* to diamond. After making the modifications indicated above, press *Apply* (to leave the *Modify plot* dialog open) or *Close* and the plot will be redrawn (above right).

You can have multiple plots open at the same time. If you don't close the plot window (by clicking the close button at the upper right border), all open plots will be closed when you exit the program. Choose *File > Print* or press the *Print* button and the plot will open in your default PDF viewer (*e.g.*, Acrobat reader). The plot can then be printed from that application. To save your plot for later modification, select *File > Save* or press the *Save* button. As noted above, you may also save your plot as a PDF or EPS file by choosing *File > Save as* or pressing the *Save as* button.

Statistical tests.

The appropriate test depends on the number of samples (two-sample and multisample tests), whether the data are categorical (observations that fall in a set of mutually exclusive categories) or measurements (*e.g.*, number of colonies, phosphorimager counts, *etc.*), and whether you are testing against an ordered alternative (one-sided) or a more general alternative hypothesis (two-sided). Most of the tests implemented in *Mstat* are summarized in the table below (the hyperlinks in the Help file will take you to the appropriate section of the notes for descriptions of the tests). Two tests not included in the table are the one-sample Goodness of Fit test and the Mantel-Haenszel test, which allows the joint analysis of multiple 2 × 2 tables. You can get interactive help on choosing the right test by selecting *Which test?* from the *Help* menu.

Statistical question	Alternative hypothesis	Two samples	Multiple samples
Difference in location, independent measurements	ordered	Wilcoxon rank sum	Jonckheere-Terpstra
	general	Wilcoxon rank sum	Kruskal-Wallis
Difference in location, paired measurements	ordered or general	Wilcoxon signed rank	
Difference in proportions, binary classification, independent samples	ordered	Fisher's exact	Cochran-Armitage
	general	Fisher's exact or Chi-square	Chi-square
Difference in proportions, binary classification, paired samples	ordered or general	McNemar	
Difference in proportions, multiple categories	general	Chi-square or partitioned LR test	Chi-square or partitioned LR test
Difference in survival (with censored data)	general	Logrank	Logrank
Correlation	ordered or general	Kendall's or Spearman's rank correlation	
Parallelism of two or more lines	ordered or general	Sen-Adichie	Sen-Adichie

In order to perform a two-sample test (*e.g.*, Wilcoxon rank sum, Wilcoxon signed rank, Kendall's rank correlation), choose the appropriate test from the *Test* menu and you will see a dialog box similar to that shown below. For our data, choose *Wilcoxon* from the *Test* menu.

The name of the test is shown in the title bar, and the two listboxes will contain all of the currently defined regular variables. Choose one variable from each listbox,

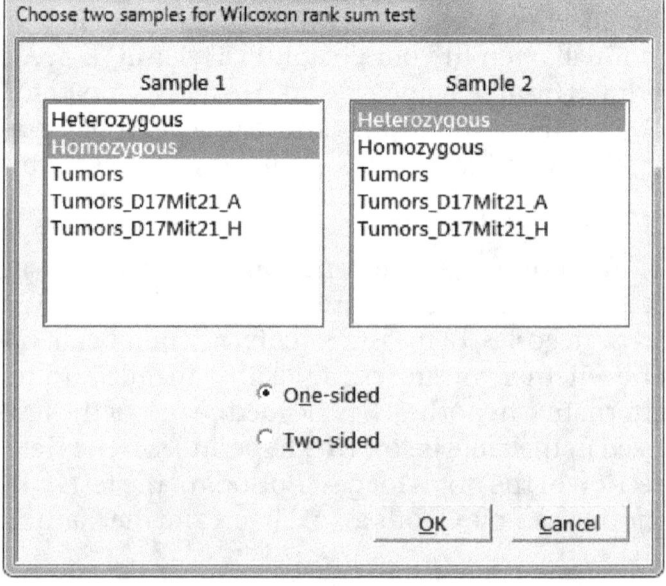

check the appropriate radiobutton for a one-sided or two-sided test, and press *OK*. The results of the test will appear in the output window.

```
Wilcoxon rank sum test
Sample        N   Mean   St. dev.
Homozygous    47  5.213  6.669
Heterozygous  50  18.1   19.53
W = 1745.5   W* = -4.044   P(one-sided) = 2.624e-5
One-sided alternative: Homozygous < Heterozygous
```

The second-last line of the output above contains the rank sum statistic, the normalized form of the statistic, and the *P*-value. The last line indicates the direction of the one-sided test that gave the *P*-value. If you had the other direction in mind (*i.e.*, Homozygous > Heterozygous), the appropriate *P*-value is the complement (1-*P*) of the value printed out.

Categorical data are stored as tables, like the TumorIncidence table we entered above. Both Fisher's exact test and the Chi-square test allow analysis for a set of one or more tables. Choose *Fisher's exact* from the *Test* menu to get the dialog box above right:

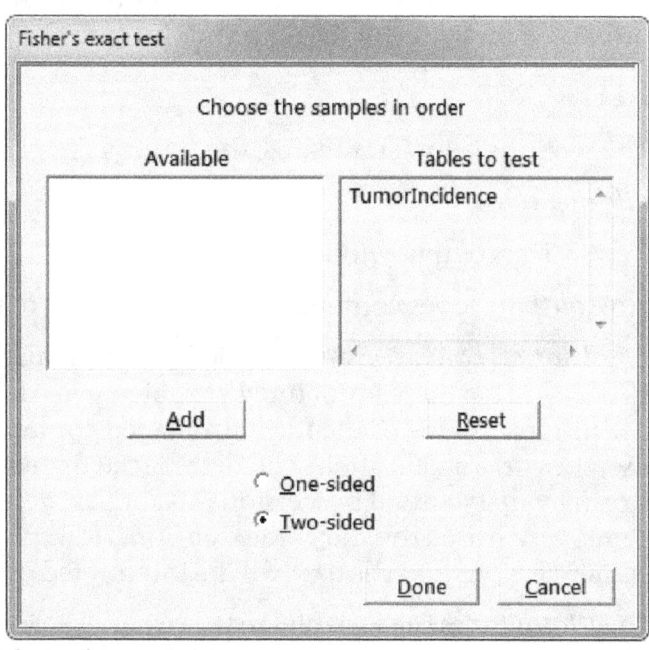

Select the desired table(s) in the *Available* box by double-clicking on each or highlight them and press the *Add* button to move them to the *Tables to test* box. Choose a one- or two-sided test by selecting the appropriate radiobutton, then press *Done*. You should see the following in the output window:

```
Fisher's exact test
Table TumorIncidence
Genotype      TumorBearing  TumorFree  Total
Homozygous    34            16         50
Heterozygous  45            2          47
Total         79            18         97
P(two-sided) = 0.0004636
```

Saving output and data files.

When you've completed a session (or periodically during lengthy data entry sessions), you can save the current data set by choosing *Save data* from the *File* menu, or pressing the *Save data* button. You will get a standard *File save* dialog. You can print the contents of the output window to the current default printer by choosing *Print* from the *File* menu (or pressing the *Print output* button) and save it to a text file by choosing *Save output* from the *File* menu. When you quit the program (choose *Exit* from the *File* menu), you will be prompted to save both the data and the output window if the files are not up to date.

REFERENCE

The sections below summarize the actions associated with each menu item.

File menu

New: Clears output window.

Save output: Saves contents of output window to text file.

Load data: Loads an *Mstat* data file (which has an ".ijd" extension) into the current session. If you have already defined variables, you will be given a chance to save the current definitions to a file. If the file to be loaded contains variable names that are already in use, the current definitions will be replaced in memory by the new data. The format for storing variables used by Version 3.0 and later differs from that used by previous versions, which used the ".jd" file extension. However, you can load data files generated by earlier versions and the data will be interpreted correctly.

Save data: Saves the variables in the current session to a data file. *Mstat* data files are text files that are J scripts beginning with the line "NB. ijd file". You can edit the file with any text editor, but probably shouldn't unless you are familiar with the J programming language. The keyboard shortcut *Ctrl-s* applies this function.

Import data: You can import data into an *Mstat* session from a tab-delimited or comma-delimited text file, such as those produced by spreadsheet programs like Microsoft Excel or OpenOffice Calc. Version 5.21 has improved the responsiveness of the import function for very large data tables and added the ability to import compressed (gzipped, extension .gz) files. See the example above in the tutorial.

Export data: Regular and indicator variables can be saved to a comma-delimited (csv) text file.

Print: Prints contents of output window to default printer. The keyboard shortcut for this function is *Ctrl-p*.

Printer setup: Choose the default printer.

Preferences: Sets program preferences through the following dialog box at right.

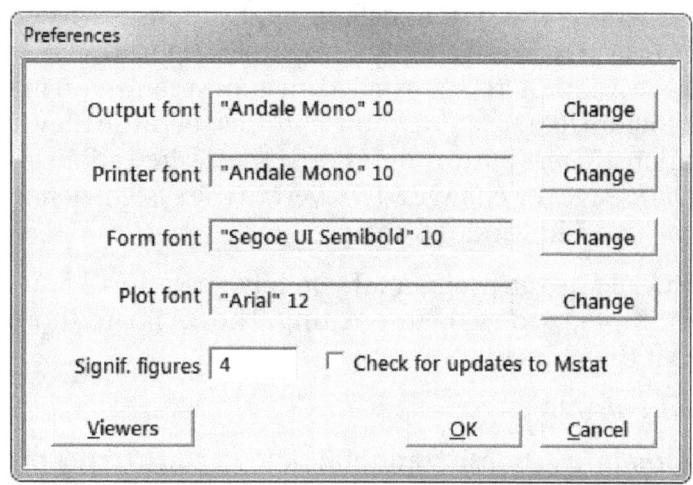

Press the appropriate *Change* button to call up a font dialog box to choose a font for the output window, the printer, or all of the program dialog boxes (*Form font*). You should select a monospaced font for the output window and printer so that tabular material lines up correctly. The "Andale Mono" font is an easy-to-read, sans serif font that was included with Internet Explorer 5, but is no longer installed by default in Windows (though it is included in OSX). You can download the font from (http://sourceforge.net/project/showfiles.php?group_id=34153). The form font is a matter of taste, but choose a size that does not result in truncation of the labels on the dialog boxes. The *Signif. figures* edit box determines the number of significant figures displayed in the output and must be between 2 and 9. Changes made through the Preferences dialog are immediately written to disk in the file "mstat6.ini" and will apply for the remainder of the current session and for subsequent sessions. Beginning with version 5.3, minor updates to *Mstat* can now be downloaded and installed automatically. To enable automatic (weekly) checking for an updated version of *Mstat*, select the checkbox in the dialog. Pressing the *Advanced* button will bring up the following dialog:

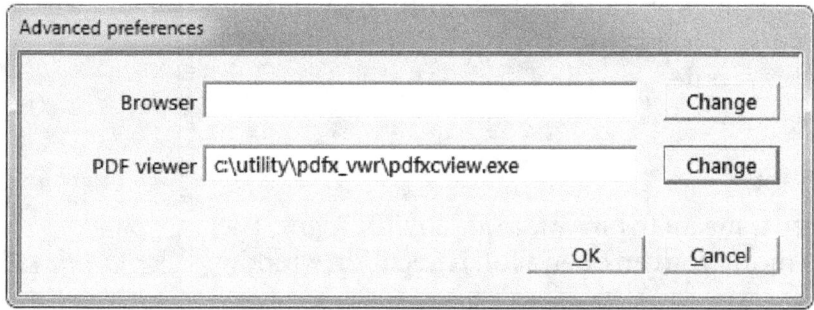

The *Browser* is used for visiting the *Mstat* website (from the *About* dialog) and, on Linux and OSX, for displaying the *Help* file. The *PDF viewer* is used for optimal printing of plots. Generally, the system default applications for these functions will be used by *Mstat*. However, you can specify alternative applications using this dialog. For example, if you have Adobe Acrobat installed on your system, you may prefer to use *Preview* on OSX or a program like *Foxit Reader* on Windows because they load more quickly. Press the appropriate *Change* button and choose the desired application from the file open dialog. Press *OK* to save the changes. To revert to the system default applications, clear the entries in the two edit windows and press *OK*.

Exit: Exits the program. If you have not already saved the data or output, you will be prompted to do so before exiting. The keyboard shortcut *Ctrl-q* (*Ctrl-d* on OS X) will also exit the program.

Edit menu

Annotate: Choosing annotate allows you to enter or edit text in the output window, so that you can make notes regarding your analyses that will be saved or printed with the rest of the output.

Undo: Available only when in annotate mode, causes the contents of the output window to revert to what it was before entering that mode.

Scratchpad: The Scratchpad allows you to perform calculations in J notation. Enter a valid J expression in the edit box, press the return key, and the results of that expression will appear in the edit window, as shown below. Press the *Reset* button to clear the edit window, the *Help* button to print a short help message to the window, or the *Done* button to dismiss the Scratchpad. A brief summary of J notation is included in the Appendix. Temporary variables may be defined in the Scratchpad and are available until the *Mstat* session is terminated. For example, to assign the vector 1 2 3 4 5 to the variable *a*, enter

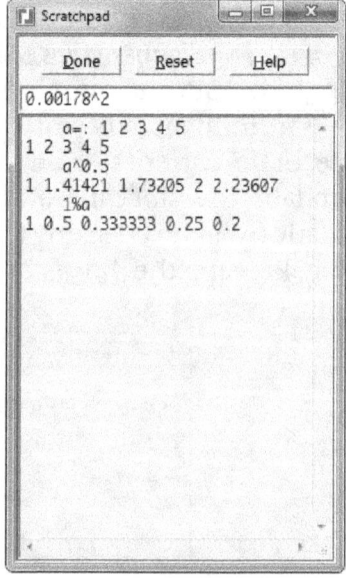

```
a=: 1 2 3 4 5
```

in the edit window.

The Scratchpad is meant to provide a safe environment. The more daring among you can open a full J execution window using *Ctrl-W*.

Data menu

New: Adds a new variable to the session; you may also use the shortcut *Ctrl-n*. See the tutorial for a discussion of this dialog window. For regular variables, the data in the edit box is evaluated as follows. The program first attempts to evaluate the contents as a list of simple numbers (*e.g.*, 2 3 –5 1e-5 assigns a list of four numbers to the variable). If that attempt fails, the portions that are not simple numbers are evaluated as J expressions. It is a good idea to enclose the J expressions in parentheses. In the dialog box below, the variable "Testvar" is assigned the list of values [1 2 3 0 0 0 0 4]. Tables or Indicator variables may be entered by choosing the appropriate radiobutton. For Indicator variables, spaces are allowed in an item as long as the item is delimited by double quotes.

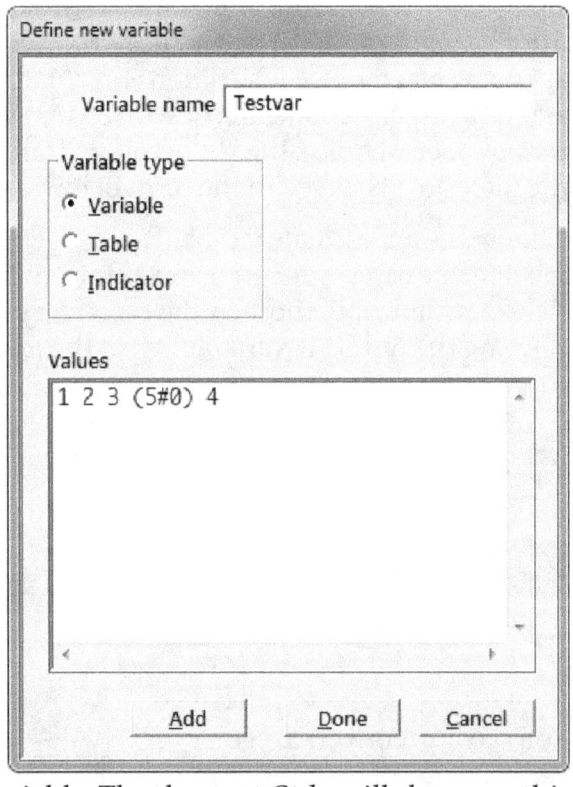

Edit: Allows you to edit the contents of a variable. The shortcut *Ctrl-e* will also open this dialog. Use of J notation is allowed in the edit window, as described for the *Data>New* entry. See the discussion in the tutorial.

Show: Prints the contents of one or more variables to the output window.

Classify: Uses an indicator variable to generate new variables consisting of a subset of the data contained in a variable. The indicator and variable must have the same number of values in the appropriate order.

Convert: The choice *Ordered table to variables* converts a table variable in which the columns follow a natural order into simple variables on a row by row basis, converting each observation in the row to a numerical value equivalent to the column number. The names of the variables are constructed as "TableName_RowName". For example, the table "hyperplasia" contains data from histological analysis of sections from animals homozygous for one of several alleles at a particular locus. Each section is evaluated and the level of hyperplasia in the tissue is graded as absent, moderate, or severe. After selecting the *Data > Convert >Ordered table to variable* menu choice, the "hyperplasia" table is chosen from the dialog box. The data in the table are displayed in the form below:

Choose the appropriate radiobutton, depending on whether the columns are in increasing or decreasing order. In our example, the observations in the first column will be assigned a value of 0, those in the second a value of 1, and those in the last a value of 2. *Show*ing the resulting variables gives the following output.

```
hyperplasia_wt
0 0 0 0 0 0 0 0 0 0 1 1 1 1 2 2 2 2

hyperplasia_m1
0 0 0 0 0 1 1 1 1 1 1 1 1 1 2 2

hyperplasia_m2
0 0 0 0 0 0 1 1 2

hyperplasia_m3
0 0 0 1 1 1 1 1 1 2 2 2 2 2 2 2 2
```

You can also convert a regular variable into an indicator variable or an indicator into a regular variable. The latter only makes sense if the indicator variable contains 'numeric' data.

Transform: Creates a new variable that is a transformation of an existing variable through the following dialog box:

Highlight the variable to be transformed in the listbox at the upper left ("Homozygous" in this case) and choose the radiobutton for the appropriate transformation. Enter an operand for the transfor-

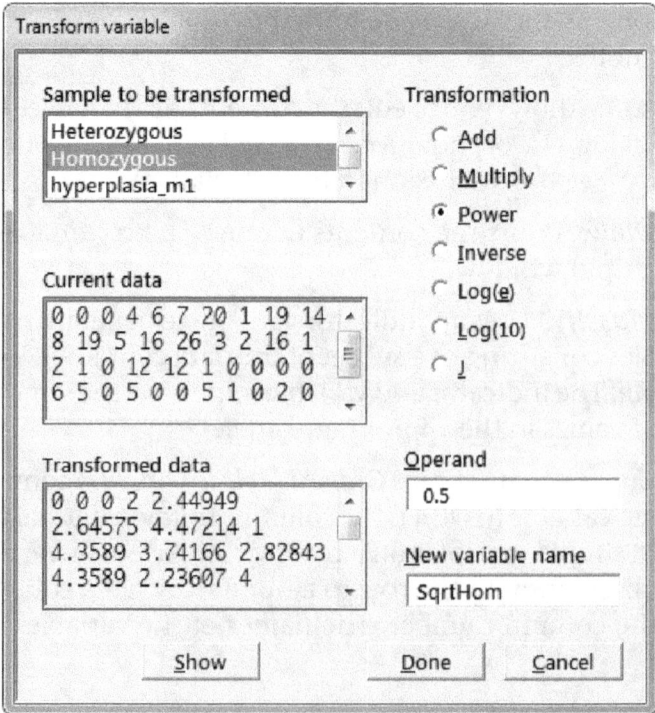

mation and a name for the new variable in the indicated edit boxes. In the example above, a new variable "SqrtHom" is being defined as the square root (0.5 power) of the variable "Homozygous". Pressing the *Show* button will display the results of the transformation; the *Done* button will enter the new variable into the current session. Note that you can easily make a copy of a variable under a new name by *Add*ing 0 or *Multiply*ing by 1. The *J* transformation allows you to enter any allowable J expression as the *Operand* to perform a functional transformation. For example, the expression ^.@(1&+) will transform the data by adding the value 1 to it and taking the natural log. The on-screen, dialog help (see below) contains other useful J phrases.

Delete: Select the variable type using the radiobuttons. Choose variables from the *Available* listbox by double-clicking or highlighting them and using the *Add* button. Pressing *Done* will delete the selected variables from memory.

Clear: Remove all variables from the current session (I hope you saved them first).

Analysis menu

Descriptive: Descriptive statistics will be printed to the output window for the set of variables chosen in the dialog box.

Bin data: Prints (and optionally plots) the sample distribution for one or more variables. Choose the desired variables from the multisample dialog and the *Bin data* dialog (above) will be displayed. The selected variables are listed in the edit box at the top of the dialog. Choose the interval type from the radiobuttons at left. If *Specify upper bounds* is chosen, enter the upper bound for each interval in the edit box at the bottom of the dialog. Parameters for equal size

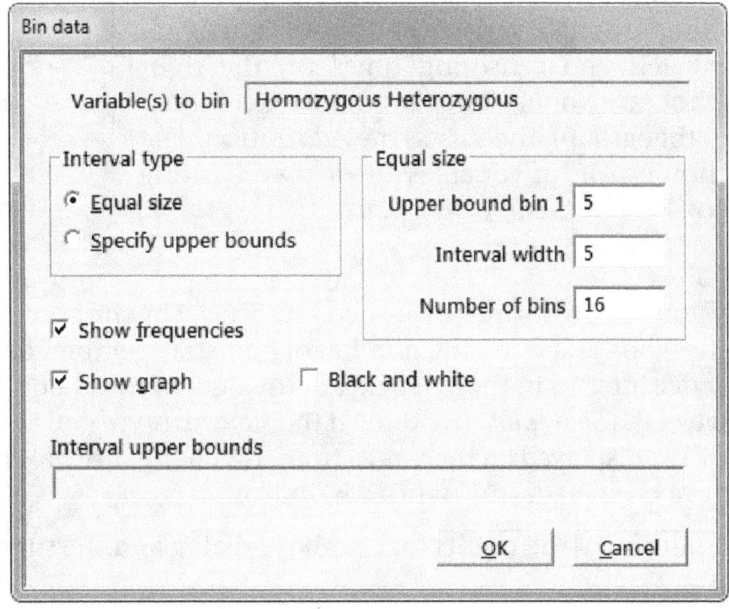

bins are entered as indicated in the group of three edit boxes. After specifying the upper bound of bin 1 and the interval width, press the *Enter* key (while the cursor is in the interval width or number of bins edit boxes); the program will suggest a number of bins such that the largest observation is placed in the second last bin. Check *Show graph* to display histograms for the binned variables. The *Black and white* option sets the plot colors to shades of gray as a starting point; all color options are available from the *Plot parameters* dialog. The number of observations in each bin is printed to the output window, along with the frequencies if *Show frequencies* is checked.

Kaplan-Meier analysis: The Kaplan-Meier (product limit) method may be used to estimate survival distributions when some of the samples are censored. For each group, the failure (or other event) times and censoring times are stored in independent variables. Choose the appropriate failure and censoring times for each group using the *Paired-sample* dialog box as shown below. The available variables are shown in the *Event times* and *Censor times* listboxes. The value "(None)" is also included at the top of the each list. For each group, select the appropriate variable for the event times on the left and censoring times on the right (choose "(None)" if no samples were censored in that group), then press the *Add* button. The chosen pairs of variables are displayed in the box labeled *Event, Censor pairs*.

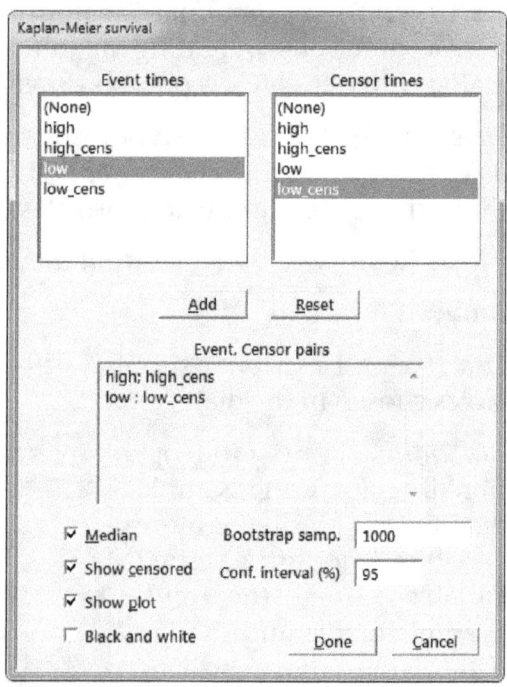

If you want to estimate the median survival by the bootstrap method, select the *Median* checkbox and enter the number of bootstrap samples desired and the size of the confidence interval in the edit boxes at the right of the dialog. To display the survival curves, select the *Show plot* checkbox. If the *Show censored* checkbox is selected, censoring times will be displayed on the plot as tic marks on the survival curves. When all of your choices have been made, press the *Done* button.

A portion of the results for the above dialog and the survival plot are shown below.

```
Kaplan-Meier survival
Events: high
Censored: high_cens
Time    Events   At risk   Survival
24      1        19        0.9474
37      2        18        0.8421
39      1        16        0.7895
40      3        15        0.6316
45      1        12        0.5789
...
69      1        5         0.2105
70      1        4         0.1579
72      1        3         0.1053
84      1        2         0.05263
Median survival (95% CI): 50 (40,68)
```

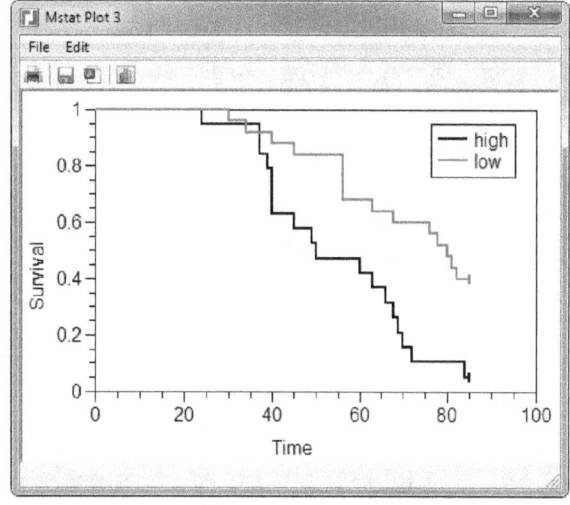

Regression: Straight line, polynomial, or multiple linear regression can be chosen from the following dialog box.

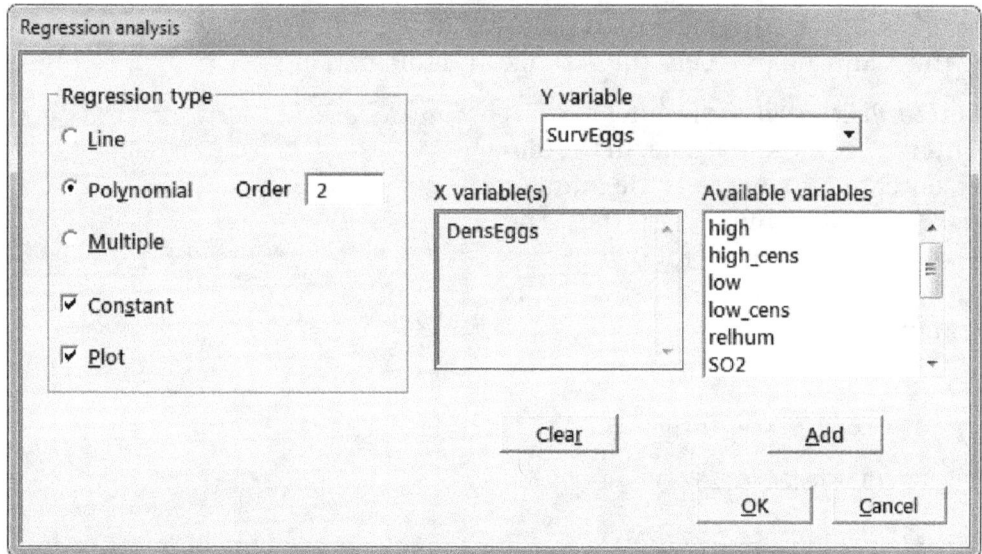

The *Y variable* is chosen from the drop box, and the *X variable(s)* are chosen from among *Available variables* by double-clicking. More than one X variable can be chosen only for the *Multiple* regression type. Checking *Constant* includes a constant term in the regression and checking *Plot* will display a plot for *Line* or *Polynomial* regression. The dialog box above generated the following output:

```
Polynomial regression, order 2
Y: SurvEggs  X: DensEggs
y = c0 + c1*X + c2*X^2

c    Parameter    std. dev.
c0        65.16        3.175
c1     -0.08048       0.1891
c2   -0.0006356     0.001756

     s2           37.16
     R2           0.7269
     N            15
```

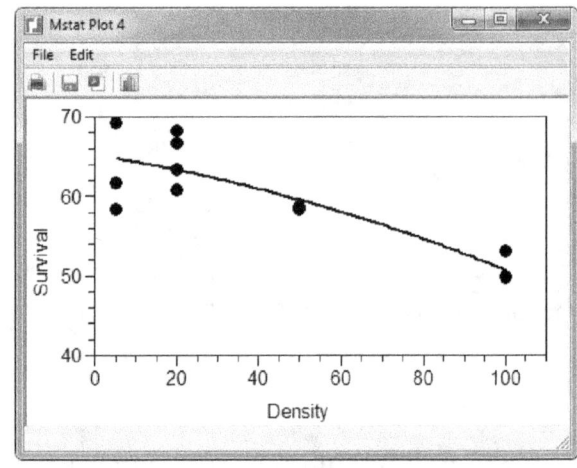

The regression equation is printed, followed by a table with the value of each parameter and its standard deviation. R2 is the correlation coefficient for the regression and N the number of data points.

The plot generated by this regression is shown above, following the use of *Modify plot* to change the X and Y axis labels, the X range and the marker size.

Binomial conf. interval: Computes a confidence interval for binomial data. In the dialog box, enter "x N" where x is the number of *successes* and N the number of trials. The dialog below generated the following output (the upper and lower confidence limits are in parentheses):

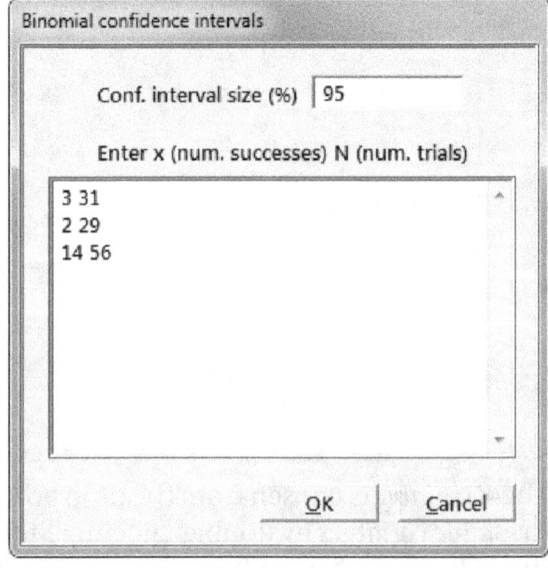

```
Binomial 95% confidence interval
x = 3, N = 31
p = 0.09677 (0.02042, 0.2575)

Binomial 95% confidence interval
x = 2, N = 29
p = 0.06897 (0.008464, 0.2277)

Binomial 95% confidence interval
x = 14, N = 56
p = 0.25 (0.1439, 0.3837)
```

Bootstrap confidence interval: Estimates a confidence interval for the mean, median, or variance of a variable using the bootstrap method. In the dialog box, choose one or more variables and enter the confidence interval size and number of bootstrap samples in the appropriate edit boxes. Choose the desired estimators (mean, median, variance) by selecting the appropriate checkboxes. A sample dialog box and the resulting output are shown below. The upper and lower confidence limits are shown in parentheses.

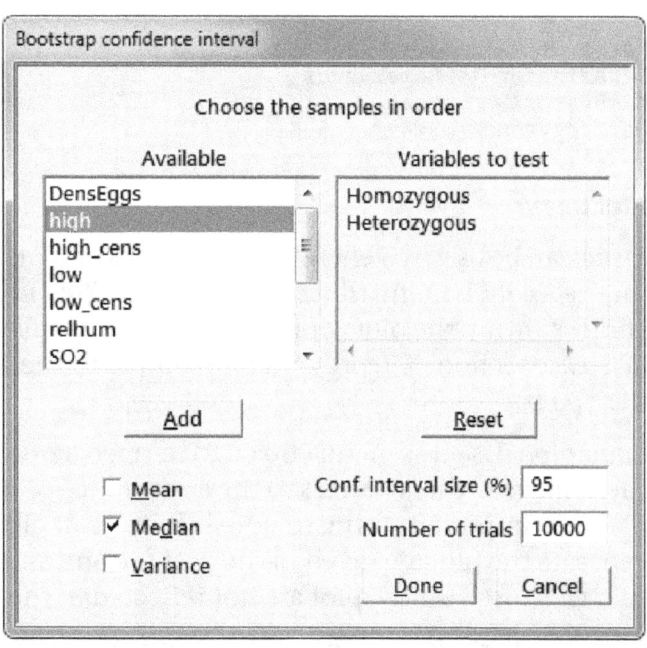

```
Bootstrap 95% confidence interval, 10000 trials
Sample: Homozygous
Median   2 (1, 5)

Bootstrap 95% confidence interval, 10000 trials
Sample: Heterozygous
Median   11 (5, 18.5)
```

Ratio: Computes the mean and standard deviation for one or more variables when taken as a ratio with another variable. This procedure is useful for reporting normalized values (*i.e.*, a value as a fraction of some control). The variable corresponding to the denominator is chosen in the lower list box. One or more variables for the numerators are chosen from among *Available* variables. The output generated is shown below.

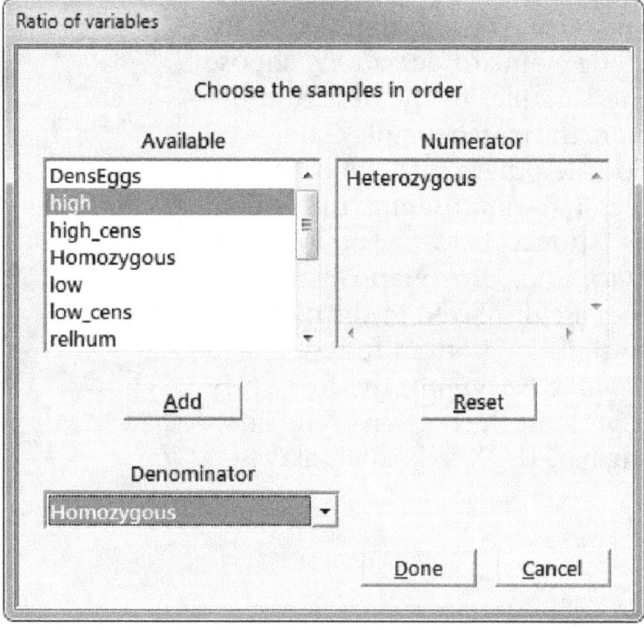

```
Ratio of variables
Denominator is Homozygous
Numerator      Mean    Std. dev.
Heterozygous   3.472   5.811
```

Plot menu

Mstat can be used to generate several types of plots in addition to those described above for the *Analysis* menu (*Bin data, Regression, Kaplan-Meier*). For a description of the menu choices within the plot window, see the section *Plot window menus* toward the end of the *Reference* section. A representative sample of the various plot types is included on the next page.

Load plot: Use this menu choice to re-open a previously saved *Mstat* plot. You can then make further changes to the appearance of the plot, or save it as a PDF or EPS file. One important thing to note is that *Mstat* plots are not "live"; the data used to generate the plot are saved in the plot file and subsequent changes to the variables that were used for the plot are not reflected in the plot window.

Dot plot: For a description of the menu choice *Dot plot*, see the tutorial.

Bar graphs: Five types of bar graphs are available from the *Plot > Bar graphs* menu choice: *Grouped, Grouped with SD, Stacked, Floating,* and *Area*. For bar graphs that include standard deviations choose the variables in the desired order from the paired sample dialog box. For the other plots, choose variables in the multisample dialog box, as shown below. For *Grouped, Stacked,* and *Area* graphs, the variables are displayed in the plot left-to-right or bottom-to-top. For a *Floating* bar graph, the first entry represents the bottom of the floating bar. The X-axis labels may be

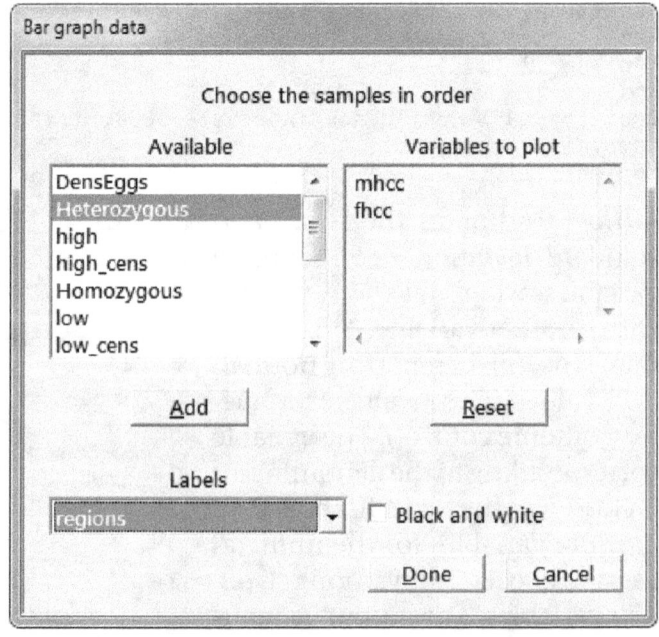

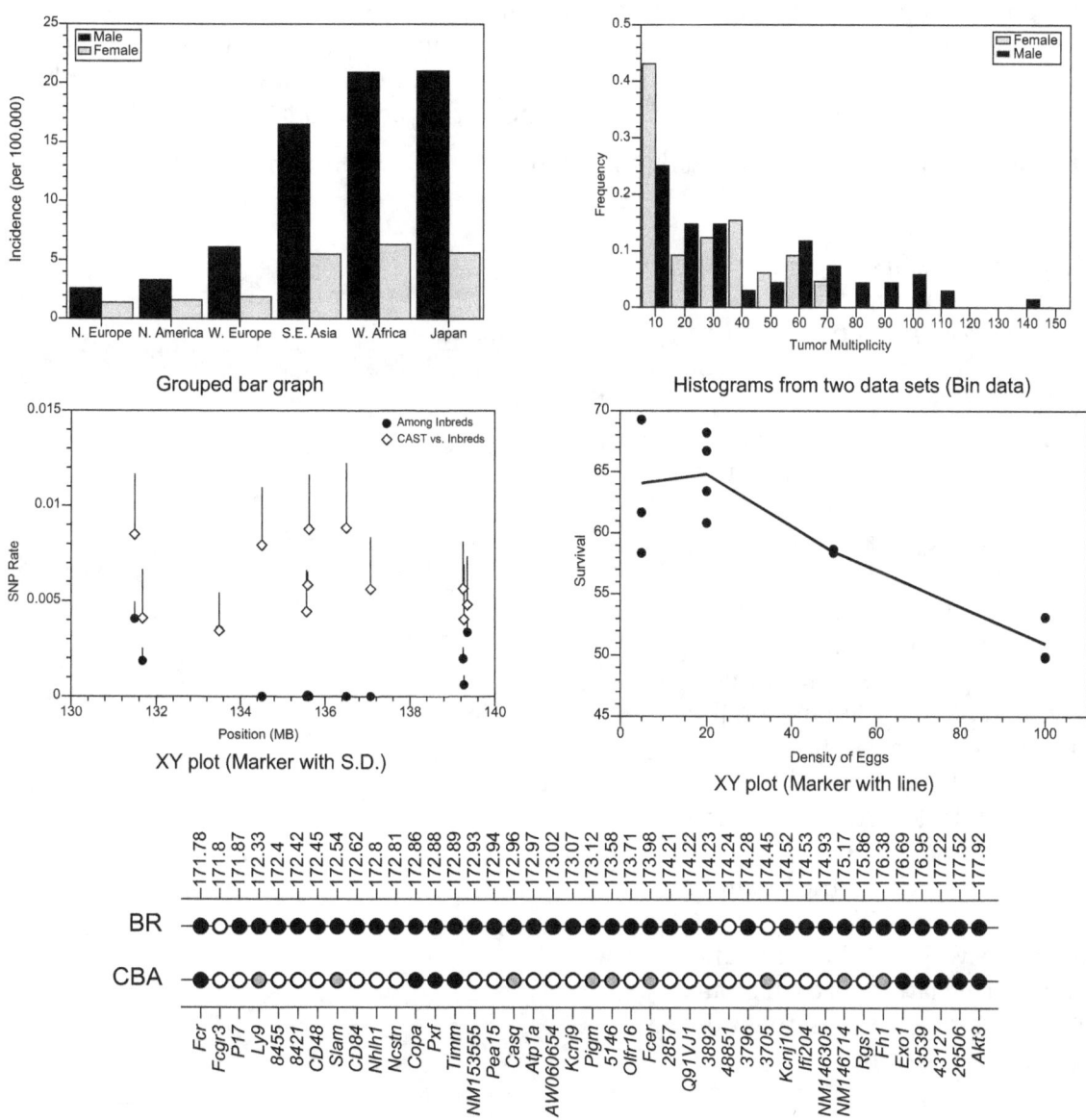

Grouped bar graph

Histograms from two data sets (Bin data)

XY plot (Marker with S.D.)

XY plot (Marker with line)

Haplotype map (made with hapmap plugin)

chosen from among the Indicator variables listed in the dropdown box at the lower left. Note that these entries may have spaces, as long as the items were delimited by quotes when the variable was defined. Each data and label variable must have the same number of values. The *Black and white* checkbox sets the initial plot colors to shades of gray.

The data from the dialog were used to generate the top-left plot on the previous page.

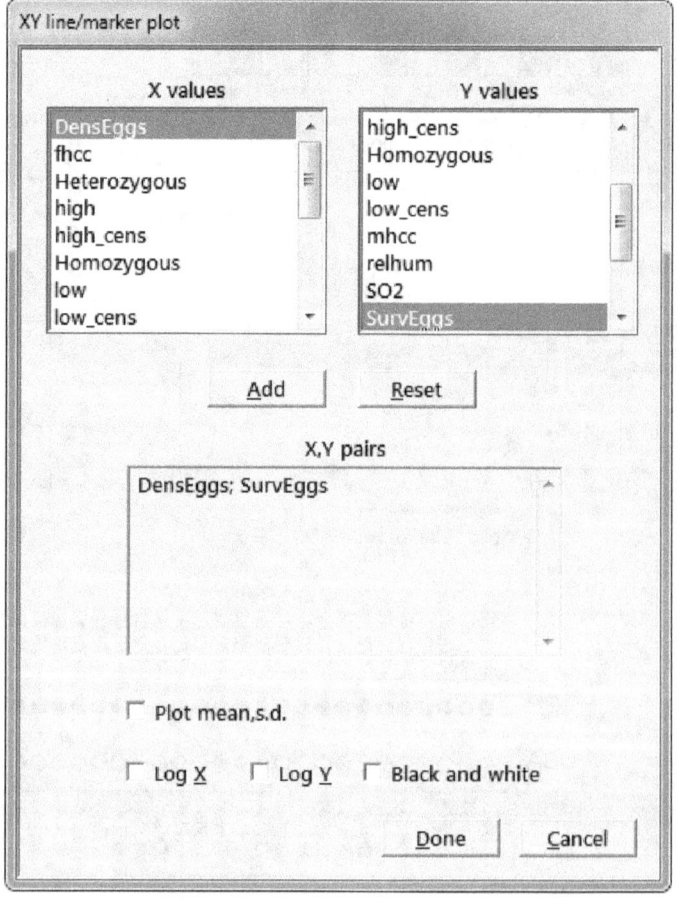

XY plots: The first three choices for this sub-menu, *Markers, Lines, Both marker/line*, can be used to generate X-Y scatter plots. For each data set, choose the X and Y values from the *Paired-sample* dialog, as shown below. Either the X or Y axis (or both) can be displayed on a log scale by selecting the appropriate check box. This choice is ignored if one or more of the data points has a value less than or equal to zero. Regardless of which plot type is chosen, the plot can later be modified to include markers, lines, or both. When multiple samples have the same X value, the line is drawn through the mean of the Y values. Selecting the *Plot mean,s.d.* checkbox will plot the mean and standard deviation for each group of X values, rather than the individual observations.

Select the *Marker with SD* choice from the *XY plots* sub-menu to plot XY data with their associated standard deviations when you have already computed the means and standard deviations. For each data set, choose the variables containing the X, Y, and SD values from the *Triplet sample* dialog as shown below.

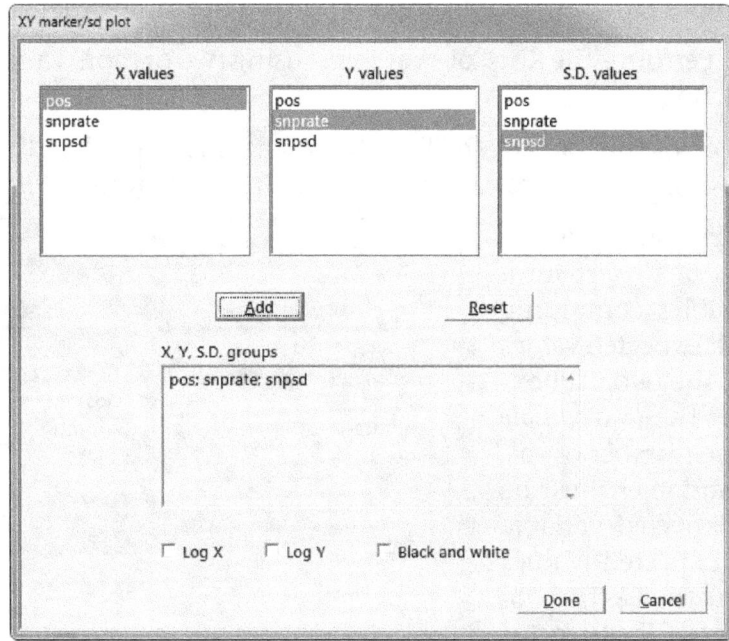

Test menu

For a complete description of each statistical test, follow the hyperlink to the corresponding section of the Notes. Choosing a test will call up a *Two-sample, Multi-sample,* or *Paired-sample* dialog box as appropriate. An example of the *Two-sample* dialog is given in the tutorial for the Wilcoxon rank sum test—select one sample in each of the two list boxes and choose the one- or two-sided radiobutton. The *Multi-sample* dialog box is similar to that shown for *Descriptive statistics* in the tutorial, except that it may contain one- and two-sided radiobuttons (or other controls) if appropriate. Select the samples in order by double-clicking in the *Available* variables list box. The selected sample will be moved over to the *Variables to test* list box. Press the *Reset* button to start over if you choose a variable by mistake. The *Paired-sample* dialog is shown above in the description of the Kaplan-Meier analysis.

Wilcoxon: Performs the Wilcoxon rank sum test using the variables selected in a *Two-sample* dialog.

Signed rank: Performs the Wilcoxon signed rank test using the variables selected in a *Two-sample* dialog. The variables, *e.g.*, "Before" and "After", must have the same number of values and should represent paired observations in the same order.

Kruskal-Wallis: Performs the Kruskal-Wallis test using two or more variables selected in a *Multi-sample* dialog.

Jonckheere: Performs the Jonckheere-Terpstra test against an ordered alternative (*e.g.*, dose response) using two or more variables chosen (in order) from a *Multi-sample* dialog.

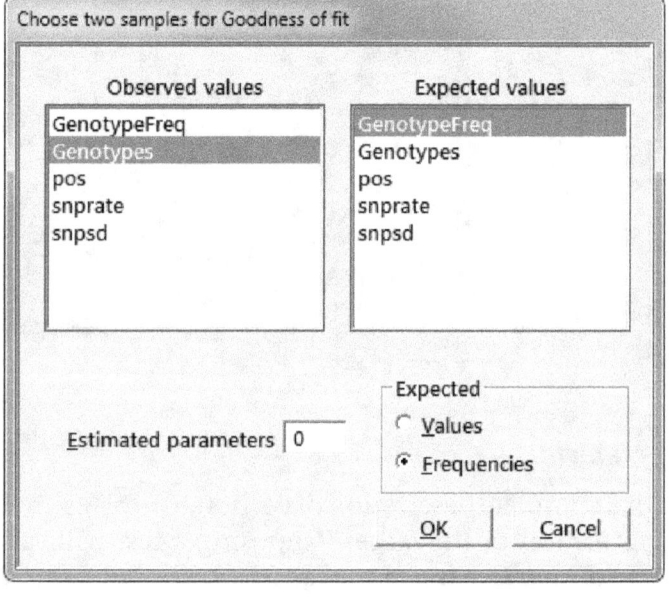

Goodness of fit: Performs the Chi-square goodness of fit test for a $1 \times c$ table. Variables containing the Observed and Expected values are chosen from the two list boxes, as indicated in the *Two-sample* dialog below. The number of values in the two variables must be identical. The Expected variable may either be Expected Values (sums to the same total as the Observed) or Expected Frequencies (sums to 1.0), with the appropriate type chosen from the radio-buttons below. The number of estimated parameters must be entered in the edit box. For example, consider the following data:

```
Genotypes
1 9 9

GenotypeFreq
0.25 0.5  0.25
```

The dialog above gave the following results.

```
Chi-square goodness of fit test
Genotypes (Observed)       1      9      9
GenotypeFreq (Expected)   4.75   9.5   4.75
X2 = 6.789 P = 0.03355 (2 degrees of freedom)
```

Fisher exact: Fisher's exact test is performed for one or more 2 × 2 tables chosen from a *Multi-sample* dialog.

Barnard exact: Barnard's exact test is performed for one or more 2 × 2 tables chosen from the dialog below.

Tables are selected as from the multi-sample dialog box. All tables must have either fixed row or column totals, which is indicated by selecting the appropriate radio button. For tables with the largest fixed total (row or column) equal to 25 or less, Barnard's CSM method is used to determine the critical region for the test (CSM-order). If either of the fixed totals exceeds 25, the critical region consists of those tables with a Fisher's exact *P*-value that does not exceed that for the observed table (F-order).

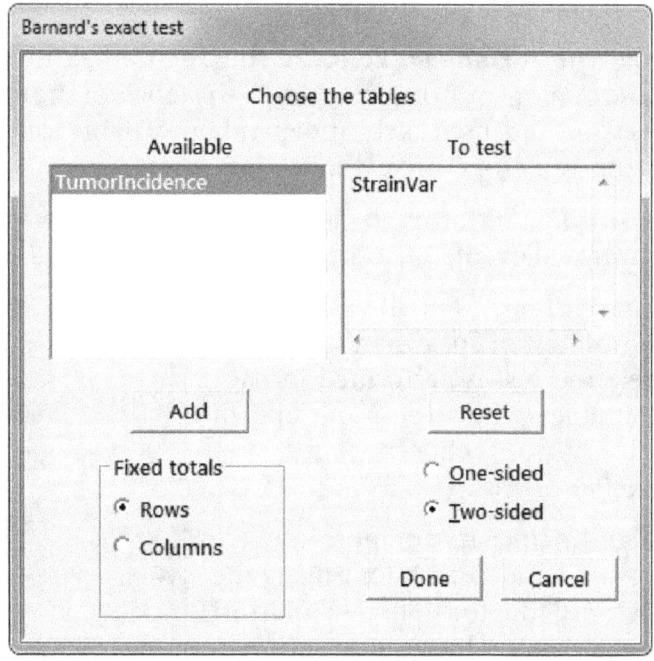

```
Barnard's exact test (CSM-order)
Table StrainVar
Fixed rows
          Tumor   Tumor-free   Total
Strain1    1         20         21
Strain2    5         12         17
Total      6         32         38
P(two-sided) = 0.04886
```

Chi-square: The Chi-Square test is performed for one or more *r* × *c* tables chosen from a *Multi-sample* dialog.

Partition table: One or more $r \times c$ tables may be selected from the *Multi-sample* dialog box. Each table is partitioned into $(r\text{-}1)(c\text{-}1)$ tests with 1 degree of freedom. Radiobuttons allow you to choose whether a Chi-square test or likelihood ratio test is performed.

McNemar: For one or more 2×2 tables consisting of paired observations, McNemar's test is performed. In addition to the *P*-value, the odds ratio and its 95% confidence limits are also reported.

Cochran-Armitage: Performs the Cochran-Armitage test for a trend in proportions for one or more $r \times 2$ or $2 \times c$ tables. If the labels of the *r* rows (or *c* columns) are numeric, these values are used as the independent variable for the regression, otherwise the integers from 1 to *r* (or *c*) are used.

Logrank: Performs the logrank test for differences in survival between two or more groups of event/censoring times chosen from a *Paired-sample* dialog.

Correlation: Kendall's rank correlation test or Spearman's rank correlation test is performed for two variables (with an equal number of observations) chosen from a *Two-sample* dialog.

Sen-Adichie: Two or more lines are tested for identical slope using the Sen-Adichie test. The X-Y pairs of variables are chosen from a *Paired-sample* dialog.

Pairwise test: This menu choice provides a convenient shortcut to performing multiple two-sample tests, including the Wilcoxon rank sum test or the Spearman or Kendall rank correlation test. For the latter two tests, all groups must have the same number of observations. Choose the relevant groups from the available list as shown below. The desired test is selected

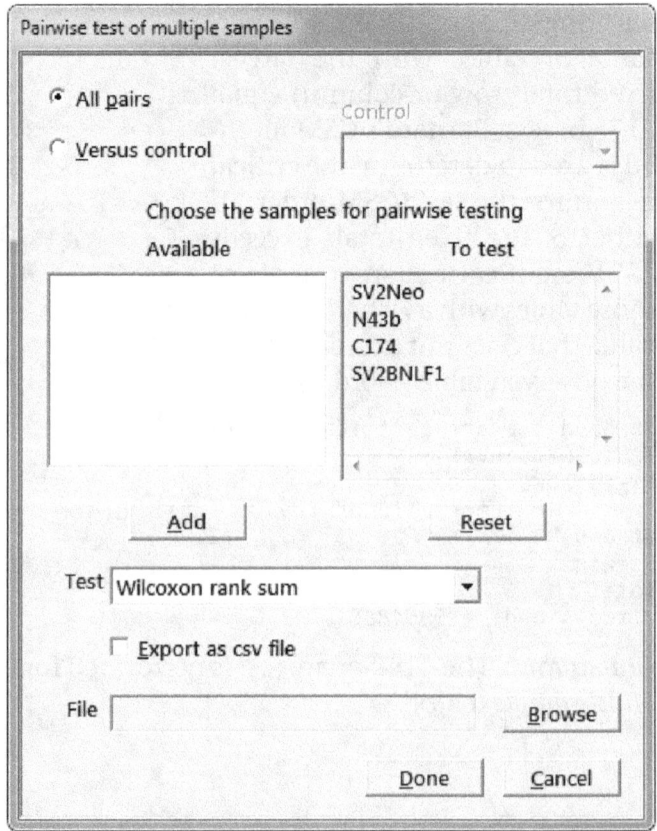

from the drop-down box below the variables. Either all pairwise tests, or each group versus a control may be tested, depending on the radiobutton selected at the top of the dialog. In the latter case, the control group is chosen from the drop-down box to the right. The results may be exported to a csv file, by selecting the checkbox and choosing a file name using the *Browse* button.

```
Pair-wise Wilcoxon rank sum tests, two-sided
Sample 1   Sample 2    W*         P-value       Bonf. P      FDR
SV2Neo     SV2BNLF1    -4.685     2.805e-6      1.683e-5     1.683e-5
N43b       SV2BNLF1    -4.04      5.343e-5      0.0003205    0.0001603
SV2Neo     C174        -3.455     0.0005509     0.003301     0.001102
N43b       C174        -3.199     0.00138       0.008249     0.002069
C174       SV2BNLF1    -1.981     0.04764       0.2539       0.05717
SV2Neo     N43b         0.3267    0.7439        0.9997       0.7439
```

Note that two-sided tests are performed for the relevant pairs. The last two columns in the output provide the Bonferroni (Dunn-Sidak) corrected *P*-value and the false discovery rate.

Multiple experiments: Perform a joint analysis of replicate experiments, each consisting of two samples, *x* and *y*. The *x,y* pairs are selected in a *Paired-sample* dialog. An exact test is done if the maximum value across the experiments of $N!/n_x!(N-n_x)!$ is less than 200,000 (where n_x is the number of *x* observations and *N* is the total number of observations in the experiment). Otherwise, Lehman's approximate test is used.

Mantel-Haenszel: A set of replicate 2×2 tables is chosen from the *Multi-sample* dialog box and tested jointly for a difference in proportions.

Combine P: Fisher's method for combining the results of statistical tests is applied to the set of *P*-values entered into the dialog box.

The *P*-values should be separated by spaces or carriage returns. The above dialog gives the output

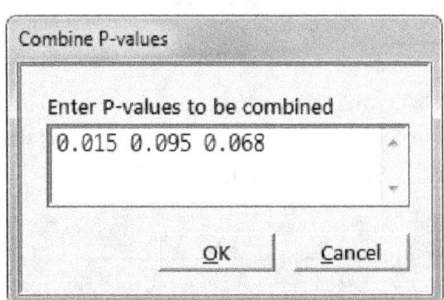

```
Fisher's method for combining P-values
P-values:  0.015 0.095 0.068
X2 = 18.48 (6 df)   P = 0.005131
```

Design menu

Distributions: For the Normal distribution, the upper or lower tail probability or the value for the cumulative distribution is output for one or more *z*-values entered into the dialog box. For the Chi-square distribution, enter the number of degrees of freedom in the upper edit box and the X^2 values in the lower edit box to output the upper tail probabilities.

For the Poisson, binomial, hypergeometric, or negative binomial distributions, the parameters of the distribution are entered into a dialog box, as shown below for the Poisson distribution. Note that three values of the Poisson parameter, m, are entered into the edit window.

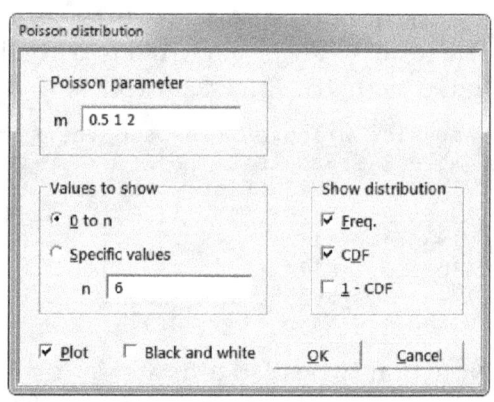

The distribution(s) from 0 to a specified value, n, in terms of the frequencies, cumulative distribution function, and/or 1-CDF, can be output for one or more distributions with the specified parameters. Alternatively, a list of frequencies for particular values of x can be output if the *Specific values* radiobutton is checked and the values entered in the edit box below. The above dialog box yields the output:

```
Poisson distribution
m = 0.5 1 2
x      f(x)                              F(x)
0      0.6065     0.3679   0.1353        0.6065 0.3679 0.1353
1      0.3033     0.3679   0.2707        0.9098 0.7358  0.406
2      0.07582    0.1839   0.2707        0.9856 0.9197 0.6767
3      0.01264    0.06131  0.1804        0.9982  0.981 0.8571
4      0.00158    0.01533  0.09022       0.9998 0.9963 0.9473
5      0.000158   0.003066 0.03609            1 0.9994 0.9834
6      1.316e-5   0.0005109 0.01203           1 0.9999 0.9955
```

Two parameters, m and k, are required for the negative binomial distribution, which has the form

$$f(x) = \left(\frac{k}{m+k}\right)^k \frac{\Gamma(k+x)}{x!\Gamma(k)} \left(\frac{m}{m+k}\right)^x$$

In this form, k may take non-integer values. An alternative form of this distribution, defined as the distribution of the number of Bernoulli trials, N, required to obtain k successes when the success probability is p, for values of $s=N-k$ is

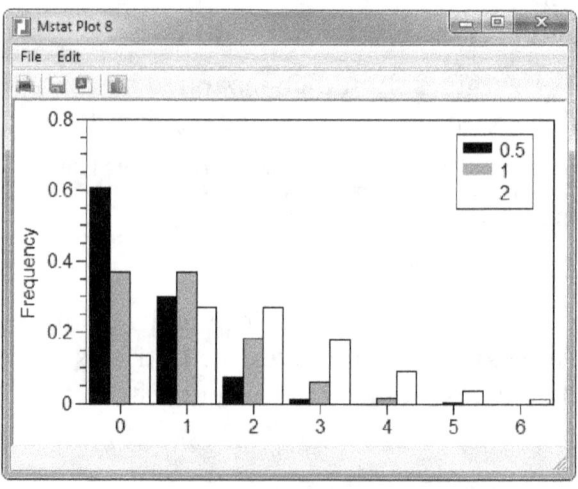

$$f(s) = \binom{k+s-1}{k-1} p^k q^s$$

In this case, the mean of the distribution (m) is rq/p, and k must be an integer.

Three parameters, N, p, and k, are required for the hypergeometric distribution. The distribution function is

$$f(x) = \frac{\binom{pN}{x}\binom{qN}{k-x}}{\binom{N}{k}}$$

A form familiar from analysis of 2×2 tables is

$$\Pr(n_{11}) = \frac{\binom{r_1}{n_{11}}\binom{r_2}{n_{21}}}{\binom{n}{c_1}} = \frac{r_1! r_2! c_1! c_2!}{n_{11}! n_{12}! n_{21}! n_{22}! n!}$$

Sample size: The sample size required for specified values of alpha (desired *P*-value) and power can be estimated for measurement variables (which would be compared by the Wilcoxon rank sum test) or proportions (for which Fisher's exact test would be used). Sample sizes for case-control studies, analyzed using McNemar's test, can also be estimated.

Parameters for the Wilcoxon rank sum test are entered into the dialog box below. The desired value of alpha, the nature of the alternative (one- or two-sided) and the power are entered in the upper part of the panel. Three alternative data models can be chosen by radiobuttons: Normal data, for which the means and variances for both groups are entered; Poisson data, which require means for the two groups; and Negative binomial data, requiring group means and a common exponent (entered in the *k* edit box). The latter model is useful when studying a *Poisson process* where the value of the Poisson parameter is itself variable. One example of this approach applied to tumor multiplicity data can be found in Drinkwater and Klotz, *Cancer Research* 41:113-119, 1981.

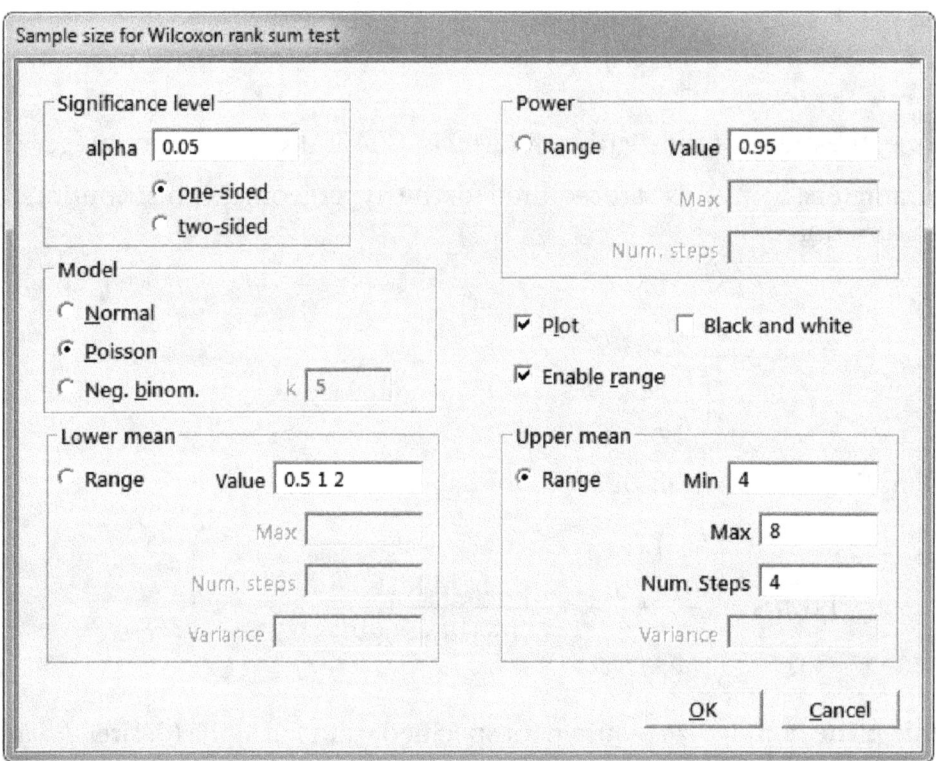

Multiple values may be entered for *Power, Lower mean,* or *Upper mean.* Only one of these three edit boxes may have multiple values, and a single value must be entered for the three edit boxes (*Min, Max, Num. steps*) for the parameter that has *Range* enabled. Filling in the values as in the above paragraph will output the necessary sample size(s) for that collection of parameters. In order to compute sample sizes for an interval of values in one of the parameters, check the *Enable range* box and select one of the three radiobuttons labeled *Range.* Edit boxes for a maximum value and number of steps in that parameter will be enabled and you can optionally plot the result. For the above dialog box, the output is

```
Sample size for Wilcoxon rank sum test.
alpha=0.05 (one-sided); Power=0.95
Poisson data, Mean(lower)=0.5 1 2
Upper Mean    N/group
4             9 11 21
5             8 9 13
6             8 8 10
7             8 8 9
8             8 8 8
```

Sample sizes for Fisher's exact test are estimated for parameters entered in a dialog box similar to the one shown above. As above, multiple values may be entered for the *Power, Lower proportion,* or *Higher proportion.*

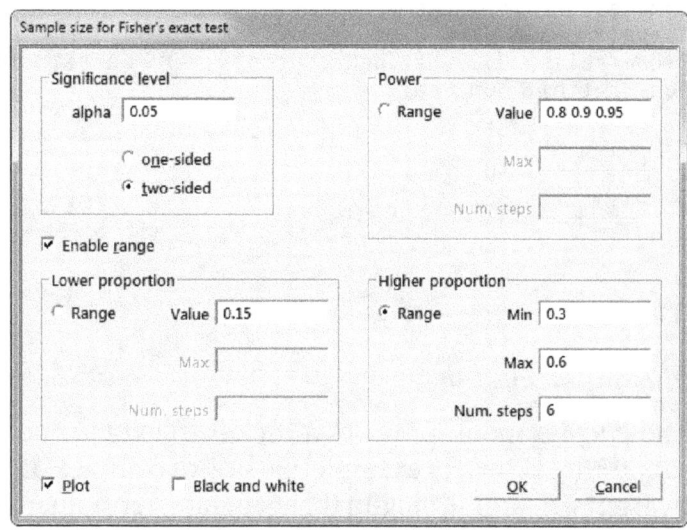

The plot generated for this set of parameters is shown below:

Sample sizes for McNemar's test are estimated by the method of Dupont (*Biometrics*, 44: 1157-1168, 1988). Values for alpha, the one- or two-sided alternative, and the power are entered into the dialog box as above. In addition to values for the probability of exposure in the control group (Control Proportion) and the odds ratio, the number of controls matched to each case and the correlation between cases and controls are entered in the remaining edit boxes. Sample output is shown below:

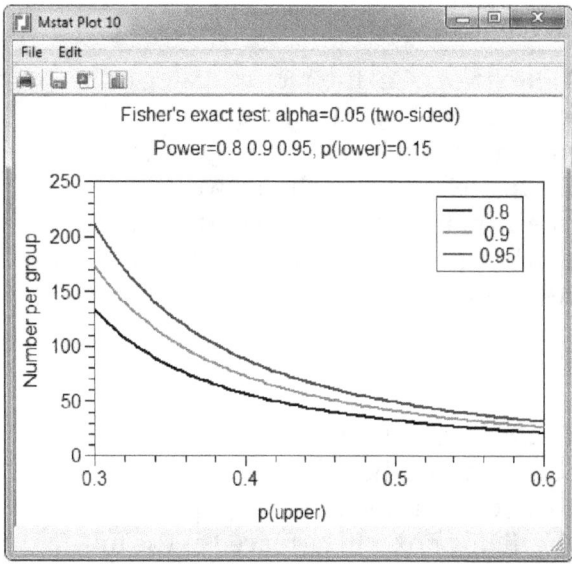

```
Sample size for McNemar's test.
Alpha(two-sided) = 0.05, Power = 0.9
P(control) = 0.2, Matched controls = 1, Correlation = 0
Odds ratio    Num. cases
2             226
3             83
4             50
5             36
6             29
7             25
8             22
9             19
10            18
```

Plug-ins menu

The *Plug-ins* menu provides a means to extend the capabilities of *Mstat* by loading J scripts that allow, for example, parsing of complex data sets or the addition of new statistical tests. A sample plug-in that generates random numbers is included in the bin\plug-in directory.

Help menu

Which test?: An interactive dialog that provides help in deciding on the appropriate statistical test. Use the drop-down box to choose the answer to each question in turn and the edit window will be filled with your choices and the recommended test as shown on the next page.

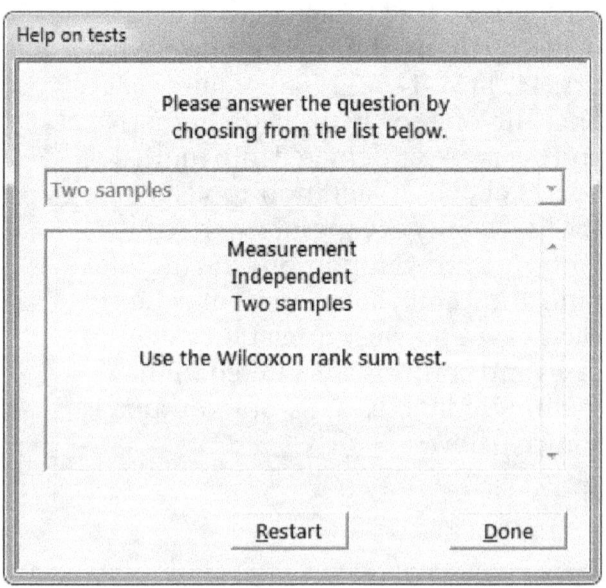

Dialog help: This menu choice toggles the dialog box help function. When activated, a window with help specific to the dialog box will be placed at the upper right of the screen. Pressing *F1* or selecting this menu item will activate or inactivate the help function. *Dialog help* can also be activated within any dialog box by pressing *Ctrl-h* (*Ctrl-l* on OS X). An example (for McNemar's test) is shown below.

Help on Mstat: Brings up the help file for *Mstat*. The F1 key will also open the help file.

Check for updates: Manually check for an updated version of *Mstat*. Version numbers for *Mstat* now have the form *x.y.z*; if the updated version is new at the *x.y* level, you will be directed to the *Mstat* website. Updates at the *z* level generally include only minor bug fixes and you will be offered the opportunity to download the new version and update the program in-place.

About: Shows a dialog with information on the program (see below). In particular, the version number and release date in this window, together with the operating system type and version, should be provided in any bug reports. Press the button on the left to check the *Mstat* website for updated software.

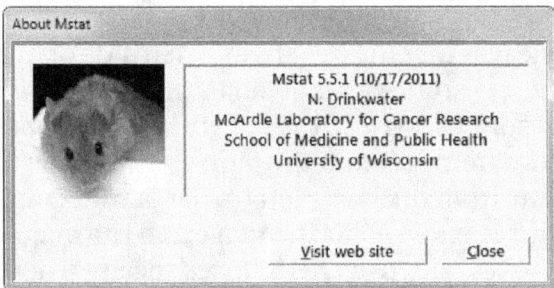

Plot window menus

The plot window contains two menus, *File* and *Edit*. Within the *File* menu, choosing *Save* will save the plot in a format (with file extension .ijg) that can be opened in a later *Mstat* session. To save the plot as a PDF or EPS file, choose *Save as* from the file menu. The resulting files may then be edited using Adobe Illustrator, the open source Inkscape drawing program, or other software. To print your plots, choose *Print* from the *File* menu. A temporary PDF file will be saved and opened in your default PDF viewer program. You can then print the plot from that program. That

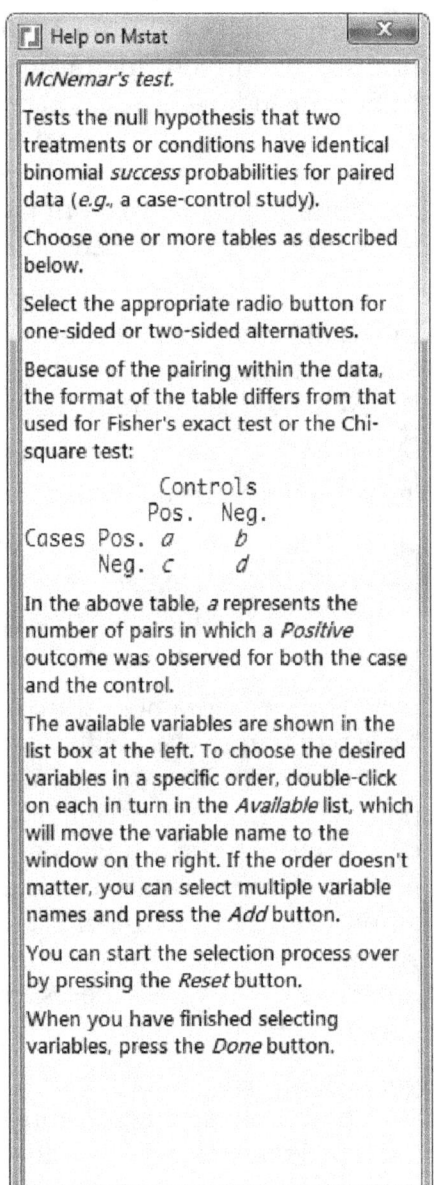

approach was chosen, rather than printing directly from the plot window to insure that the printed plots look identical on all platforms. Note that for PDF and EPS versions of the files, including the temporary file generated for printing, all fonts in the plot window are replaced with Helvetica. You should use Arial or Helvetica as the default plot face to insure that the appearance on screen matches that for the printed page. The reason for this limitation is that the font metrics for Helvetica are embedded in the program and used to generate the PDF and EPS files.

The *Edit* menu contains two choices, *Copy* and *Modify plot*. Selecting *Copy*, or pressing Ctrl-w, will copy the plot window to the clipboard. You can then paste the plot into, for example, a *PowerPoint* slide. The *Modify plot* choice will bring up a tabbed dialog allowing you to change many features of the plot. Examples for each of the four tabs are shown below.

The contents of the tabs will vary depending on the type of plot.

Labels: The larger edit fields in this tab allow you to modify the text shown for the plot title and X and Y axis captions. For bar graphs and dot plots, an additional field (*Group names*) is shown for the X axis labels; quote any entries with embedded spaces. The font sizes for each type of label may be entered in the smaller, *Size* edit boxes.

Axes: The *Tic style* radiobuttons determine whether the tics are shown inside or outside of the plot frame. The weight of the frame, axes, and tics is given in the *Line weight* edit box, and the lengths of the major and minor tics in *Tic size major* and *Tic size minor*, respectively. Checking the *Frame* box places a frame around the plot; checking the *Offset* box will move the axis origins slightly away from the lower left corner of the frame. For each axis, you can enter the minimum and maximum for the range and the major and minor tic intervals in the indicated edit boxes. The two check boxes specify whether a grid (faint lines at the major tic intervals) or log axis is shown. The *Log* check box is disabled if any of the values are less than or equal to zero. Only the Y axis is shown for dot plots or any of the bar graph types.

Symbols: An edit box for *Line weight* is shown for any of the XY plots, Kaplan-Meier plots, power plots, or regression analyses. A *Marker size* edit box is available for the XY plot types, regression plots, and dot plots. The *Marker with SD* plot type will also have a set of radiobuttons allowing you to specify whether the vertical bar indicating the standard deviation is shown above, below, or above and below the marker. The remainder of the tab consists of a table with an entry for each plotted variable. For each variable, you may set the color for the markers, lines, or bars from the 22 entries in the dropdown listbox. For plots with markers, choose from among *circle, diamond, square, triangle, plus,*

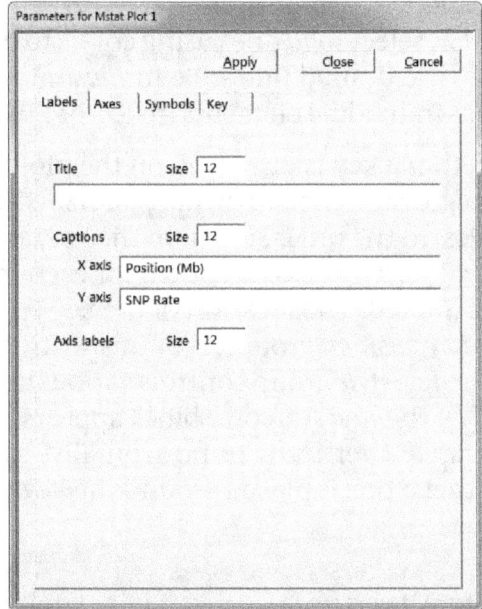

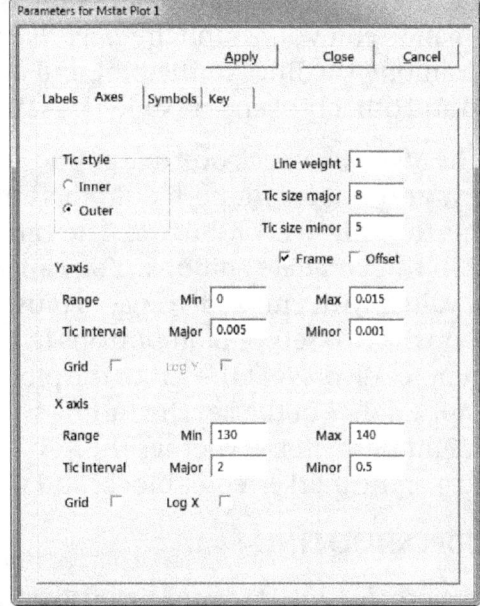

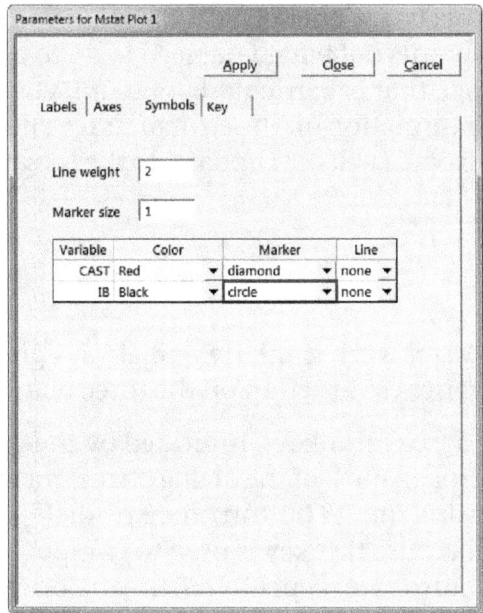

times, *vbar* (vertical bar), *opencircle*, *opendiamond*, *opensquare*, *opentriangle*, or *none*. Choices for plots with lines include *none, solid, dash, dot*, '-.' (dash-dot), and '-..' (dash-dot-dot). If you plan to edit your graph in *Adobe Illustrator*, select *solid* lines using colors to differentiate among the lines in the plot and apply the desired line style in *Illustrator*. The dashed and other broken line styles are saved as individual elements in PDF or EPS files.

Key: The *Show key* check box determines whether a key is displayed on the plot. Note that keys are disabled for both dot plots and regression plots. The *Key font size* edit box contains the font size for the text. The variables, in the order shown in the key, are displayed in the *Variables* edit box. You can specify the text to be shown for each in *Key names*; values with embedded spaces must be quoted. The location of the key is determined by the two sets of radiobuttons in the *Key position* group. As of this writing, the *Center* choice displays at the left of the plot. The *Key style* group controls various aspects of the appearance of the key, including whether the marker/color block appears to the left or right of the text, whether the key is arranged vertically or horizontally, the appearance of the marker/color block, and whether a box is placed around the key.

TROUBLESHOOTING

This version of *Mstat* was tested extensively before it was released, but it is inevitable that one or more bugs lie hidden in its 12,000 lines of code. Generally, the data that you enter are checked for validity and an error message points out what you need to do to correct the error. If, however, you see an error message that is particularly obscure, you have probably found a bug. Please write down the information on the error message and send it to me by email at drinkwater@oncology.wisc.edu. I will post updates to the program at the website

http://mcardle.oncology.wisc.edu/mstat.

Mac OS X/Linux specifics

The Windows, OS X, and Linux versions of *Mstat* work similarly and always give the same answers, but there are some minor differences in function on the three platforms.

- The Windows and Linux versions use accelerator keys, indicated by the underlined character in the label for the control, in most of the dialog boxes. For example, pressing *Alt-O* is equivalent to pressing the *OK* button on many dialogs. Alt-accelerator keys are disabled on OS X because this key is used to compose non-ascii characters. As an alternative, any buttons (except *Cancel*) in a dialog may be activated by pressing the Ctrl-key together with the first letter on the button label, except where that letter is "C", in which case you should use the second letter. The *Cancel* button can invoked using the escape key. The *Ctrl* hotkeys (*e.g.*, *Ctrl-N* invokes the *New variable* dialog) work on all operating systems, but must be activated using the *Command* key on OS X for any window with a menu.

- Although all of the files (including data, initialization, and output) used by *Mstat* are simple text files, the strict file typing imposed by some Mac programs obscures this fact. Output files can be opened by word processors by choosing the *All files* option in the file open dialog box.

- On OS X, the left-most menu (labeled *Mstat*) does not behave as expected. For example, *Mstat>About* will give a generic Java message and you should use *Help>About* to view the *Mstat* About box. In particular, do not choose *Mstat>Quit* (*Command*-Q), which will exit the program without giving you the opportunity to save your data or output. Use the *File>Exit* (*Ctrl*-Q) instead.

- The menu choice *Help > Help on Mstat* will bring up the program documentation on all operating systems. Help files on OS X and Linux are loaded in your default browser. Windows help files are viewed with the HTMLHelp program.

- Information may be copied or cut from, or pasted into, most dialogs. To access this feature, the right mouse button is used on the Windows platform while the conventional key combinations are used on OS X and Linux.

Licensing

Subject to the restrictions listed below, this software may be freely copied and used by students, faculty, and staff at academic or other non-profit research institutions. While this software is free, donations to the McArdle Laboratory for Cancer Research (1400 University Avenue, Madison, WI 53706) would be welcomed; such funds will be used to support graduate training in cancer research at the Laboratory. Commercial use of the software is prohibited without prior arrangements being made with the author.

Restrictions

1. The *Mstat* package (the software and its documentation) are copyrighted by Norman Drinkwater. The StatNotes reference material is copyrighted by Norman Drinkwater and Carter Denniston.

2. The J executable and related portions of the package are copyrighted by JSoftware, Inc.

3. This software requires the zlib library (included in the Windows distribution), which is copyrighted by Jean-loup Gailly and Mark Adler. The Windows distribution also includes the wget executable, which is subject to the GNU GPL.

4. Some toolbar icons are from the Fugue icon set and are copyrighted by Yusuke Kamiyamane and licensed under a Creative Commons Attribution 3.0 license.

5. No part of the package may be modified or used to create derivative works.

6. Use of the software should be acknowledged in any resulting publications.

7. This package is provided *as-is* and neither the author nor the University of Wisconsin is responsible for any damages resulting from its use.

Acknowledgments

I am grateful to my colleagues Rebecca Baus, Andrea Bilger, Jamie Bugni, Rey Carabeo, Teresa Chiaverotti, Brad Clark, Jennifer Drew, Mara Feld, Matt Gigot, Tonia Jorgenson, Sean McDermott, Amy Moser, Chris Oberley, Stephanie Peychal, Therese Poole, Rachel Potempa, Sue Schadewald, and Bret Williams, as well as several generations of Oncology 675/Genetics 677 students, for their help in testing the software in this and its earlier versions and for many suggestions regarding new features and usability.

Contacting the Author

Bug reports or other comments should be directed to Norman Drinkwater (drinkwater@oncology.wisc.edu). Please indicate the version of the software that you are using (provided in the *About box*).

Appendix: J Notation

A brief summary of J notation is provided below to assist in the use of the Scratchpad or the extended data entry feature for variables. For more details regarding J, see the J Software website (http://www.jsoftware.com).

Expressions in J are evaluated strictly from right to left, but parentheses can be used to alter the order of evaluation. For example, 5*3+2 gives 25, while (5*3)+2 is 17.

Negative numbers are preceded by an underscore.

Functions in J generally operate on lists of numbers as they do on single values. If one operand is a vector of length n, the other operand must be either of the same length or a scalar value. For example, if the variable x and y are assigned the values

```
        x=: 1 2 3 4 5
        y=: 1 0 1 1 0
```

then

```
        x*2
2  4  6  8  10
        x*y
1  0  3  4  0
```

The primitive J functions consist of one or two characters, as indicated in the table below for a few of the J functions likely to be most useful to you. In each definition, the meaning of the symbol is given for the monadic (symbol x) and dyadic (x symbol y) cases. The symbol →, below, indicates the result of the expression on the left.

Symbol	Function		
	Monadic	Dyadic	Examples
+		addition	3+2 → 5
-	negate	subtraction	-2 → _2 5-2 → 3
*	sign	multiplication	3*2 → 6 *_3 → _1
%	inverse	division	%2 → 0.5 8%4 → 2
^	exponential	power	^1 → 2.71828 3^2 → 9
^.	natural log	logarithm	^.2 → 0.6931 10^.2→ 0.301
=		equals	5 = 5 → 1
<		less than	1<2 → 1
>		greater than	1>2 → 0
<.	floor	lesser of	<. 1.23 → 1 2 <. 3 → 2
>.	ceiling	greater of	>. 1.23 → 2 2 >. 3 → 3
*.		and	1 *. 0 → 0
+.		or	1 +. 0 → 1
!	factorial	out of	!3 → 6 3 ! 6 → 20
#	tally	copy	# 5 6 7 → 3 3#2 → 2 2 2

REFERENCES

Adichie, J.N., 1975. On the use of ranks for testing the coincidence of several regression lines. *Annals of Statistics*, 3: 521-527.

Agresti, A., 2002. *Categorical data analysis*, 2nd ed. Hoboken: Wiley.

Agresti, A., 2007. *An introduction to categorical data analysis*, 2nd ed. Hoboken: Wiley.

Armitage, P., 1955. Tests for linear trends in proportions and frequencies. *Biometrics*, 11: 375-386.

Baichwal, V.R., & Sugden, B., 1989. The multiple membrane-spanning segments of the BNLF-1 oncogene from Epstein-Barr virus are required for transformation. *Oncogene*, 4: 67-74.

Barnard, G.A., 1947. Significance tests for 2 × 2 tables. *Biometrika*, 34: 123-138.

Benjamini, Y., & Hochberg, Y., 1995. Controlling the false discovery rate: a practical and powerful approach to multiple testing. *Journal of the Royal Statistical Society, Series B*, 57: 289-300.

Bilger, A., Bennett, L.M., Carabeo, R.A., Chiaverotti, T.A., Dvorak, C., Liss, K.M., Schadewald, S.A., Pitot, H.C., & Drinkwater, N.R., 2004. a potent modifier of liver cancer risk on distal mouse chromosome 1: linkage analysis and characterization of congenic lines. *Genetics*, 167: 859-866.

Casagrande, J.T., Pike, M.C., & Smith, P.G., 1978. An improved approximate formula for calculating sample sizes for comparing two binomial distributions. *Biometrics*, 34: 483-486.

Churchill, G.A., & Doerge, R.W., 1994. Empirical threshold values for quantitative trait mapping. *Genetics*, 138: 963-971.

Cochran, W.G., 1954. Some methods for strengthening the common chi-square tests. *Biometrics*, 10: 417-451.

Conover, W.J., 1999. *Practical nonparametric statistics*, 3rd ed. New York: Wiley.

Cox, D.R., & Oakes, D., 1984. *Analysis of survival data*. Boca Raton: Chapman & Hall/CRC.

Drinkwater, N. R., & Klotz, J. H., 1981. Statistical methods for the analysis of tumor multiplicity data. *Cancer Research*, 41: 113-119.

Dupont, W.D., 1988. Power calculations for matched case-control studies. *Biometrics*, 44: 1157-1168.

Efron, B., & Tibshirani, R.J., 1993. *An introduction to the bootstrap*. Boca Raton: Chapman & Hall/CRC.

Efron, B., 1979. Bootstrap methods: another look at the jackknife. *Annals of Statistics*, 7: 1-26.

Efron, B., 1981. Censored data and the bootstrap. *Journal of the American Statistical Association*, 76: 312-319.

Fisher, R.A., 1973. *Statistical methods for research workers*, 14th ed. New York: Hafner.

Hollander, M., & Wolfe, D.A., 1999. *Nonparametric statistical methods*, 2nd ed. New York: Wiley.

Jonckheere, A.R., 1954. A distribution-free k-sample test against ordered alternatives. *Biometrika*, 4: 133-145.

Kaplan, E.L., & Meier, P., 1958. Nonparametric estimation from incomplete observations. *Journal of the American Statistical Association*, 53: 457-481.

Kempthorne, O., 1979. In dispraise of the exact test: reactions. *Journal of Statistical Planning and Inference*, 3: 199-213.

Kendall, M.G., 1938. A new measure of rank correlation. *Biometrika*, 30: 81-93.

Kruskal, W.H., & Wallis, W.A., 1952. Use of ranks in one-criterion variance analysis. *J. American Stat. Assoc.*, 47: 583-621.

Lee, E.T., & Wang, J.W., 2003. *Statistical methods for survival data analysis*, 3rd ed. Hoboken: Wiley.

Lee, G.H., & Drinkwater, N.R., 1995. Hepatocarcinogenesis in BXH recombinant inbred strains of mice: analysis of diverse phenotypic effects of the hepatocarcinogen sensitivity loci. *Molecular Carcinogenesis*, 14: 190-197.

Lehman, E.L., 1993. The Fisher, Neyman-Pearson theories of testing hypotheses: one theory or two? *Journal American Statistical Association*, 88: 1242-1249.

Lehman, E.L., 1998. *Nonparametrics: statistical methods based on ranks*, 1st ed. revised. Upper Saddle River: Prentice Hall.

Lystig, T.C., 2003. Adjusted P values for genome-wide scans. *Genetics*, 164: 1683-1687.

Manly, B.F.J., 2001. *Randomization, bootstrap, and Monte Carlo methods in biology*, 2 ed. Boca Raton: Chapman & Hall/CRC.

Mann, H.B., & Whitney, D.R., 1947. On a test of whether one of two random variables is stochastically larger than the other. *Annals of Mathematical Statistics*, 18: 50-60.

Mantel, N., & Haenszel, W., 1959. Statistical aspects of the analysis of data from retrospective studies of disease. *Journal of the National Cancer Institute*, 22: 719-748.

Martín Andrés, A., & Silva Mato, A., 1994. Choosing the optimal unconditioned test for comparing two independent proportions. *Computational Statistics & Data Analysis*, 17: 555-574.

Martín Andrés, A., Silva Mato, A., Tapia García, J.M., Sánchez Quevedo, M.J., 2004. Comparing the asymptotic power of exact tests in 2 × 2 tables. *Computational Statistics & Data Analysis*, 47: 745-756.

McNemar, Q., 1947. Note on the sampling error of the difference between correlated proportions or percentages. *Psychometrika*, 12: 153-157.

Radelet, M.L., & Pierce, G.L., 1991. Choosing those who will die: race and the death penalty in Florida. *Florida Law Review*, 43: 1-34.

Perneger, T.V., 1998. What's wrong with Bonferroni adjustments. *British Medical Journal*, 316: 1236-1238.

Peto, R., & Peto, J., 1972. Asymptotically efficient rank invariant test procedures. *Journal of the Royal Statistical Society, Series A*, 135: 185-207.

Sen, P.K., 1969. On a class of rank order tests for the parallelism of several regression lines. *Annals of Mathematical Statistics*, 40: 1668-1683.

Smyth, G.K., 2004. Linear models and empirical Bayes methods for assessing differential expression in microarray experiments. *Statistical Applications in Genetics and Molecular Biology* **3**, No. 1, Article 3.

Sokal, R.R., & Rohlf, F.J., 1995. *Biometry: the principles and practice of statistics in biological research*, 3rd ed. New York: W.H. Freeman.

Spearman, C., 1904. The proof and measurement of association between two things. *American Journal of Psychology*, 15: 72-101.

Storer, B.E., & Kim, C., 1990. Exact properties of some exact test statistics for comparing two binomial proportions. *Journal of the American Statistical Association*, 85: 146-155.

Storey, J.D., 2002. A direct approach to false discovery rates. *Journal of the Royal Statistical Society, Series B*, 64: 479-498.

Storey, J.D., & Tibshirani, R., 2003. Statistical significance for genomewide studies. *Proceedings of the National Academy of Sciences*, 100: 9440-9445.

Sugden, B., & Metzenberg, S., 1983. Characterization of an antigen whose cell surface expression is induced by infection with Epstein-Barr virus. *Journal of Virology*, 46: 800-807.

Suissa, S., & Shuster, J.J., 1985. Exact unconditional sample sizes for the 2 × 2 binomial trial. *Journal of the Royal Statistical Society, Series A*, 148: 317-327.

Tessier, C.R., Doyle, G.A., Clark, B.A., Pitot, H.C., & Ross, J., 2004. Mammary tumor induction in transgenic mice expressing an RNA-binding protein. *Cancer Research*, 64: 209-215.

Ury, H.K., 1976. A comparison of four procedures for multiple comparisons among means (pairwise contrasts) for arbitrary sample sizes. *Technometrics*, 18: 89-97.

Wilcoxon, F., 1945. Individual comparisons by ranking methods. *Biometrics Bulletin*, 1: 80-83.

INDEX

About the authors

Dr. Norman Drinkwater is Professor of Oncology at the University of Wisconsin School of Medicine and Public Health. He served as Chair of Oncology and Director of the McArdle Laboratory for Cancer Research from 1992-2008. His research focuses on the experimental genetics of cancer risk.

Dr. Carter Denniston was Professor Emeritus of Medical Genetics at the University of Wisconsin when he died at the age of 67 in 2005. During his 35 year career on the faculty, he served as Chair of the Departments of Genetics and Medical Genetics for 7 years and did groundbreaking research in theoretical population genetics.

www.ingramcontent.com/pod-product-compliance
Lightning Source LLC
Chambersburg PA
CBHW081433170526
45166CB00008B/2198